Fundamentals of Virtual Colonoscopy

Abraham H. Dachman, MD
Professor of Radiology, The University of Chicago Medical
Center, Chicago, Illinois

Editor

Fundamentals of Virtual Colonoscopy

With 42 Illustrations in 78 Parts, 13 in Full Color

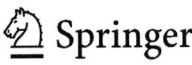 Springer

Abraham H. Dachman, MD
Professor of Radiology
The University of Chicago Medical Center
Chicago, IL 60637-1470, USA

ISBN 0-387-21912-9   Printed on acid-free paper.

Printed in the United States of America.   (MP/EB)

9 8 7 6 5 4 3 2 1   SPIN 10994900

springeronline.com

To my wife, Yisraela
and to Toby, Yitzchak, Laya, and Eliana.

In memory of my father, Albert and
my mother, Esther Deborah Dachman

Preface

It is my pleasure to present the "fundamentals" version of *Atlas of Virtual Colonoscopy,* which was first published in 2003 in two parts. The first, which is reprinted here, consists of nine expertly authored chapters that serve as an educational module and reference for a rapid review of critical areas of study. Scientific advances in research, particularly the publication of clinical trials and the gradual acceptance of virtual colonoscopy in nonresearch settings, have created a demand for this information. Yet only limited educational venues are available for those seeking courses, tutorials, and published study material. The atlas from which these chapters are derived, remains the only text of its kind on the topic, and in spite of advances since initial publication, its content remains largely up to date and relevant. This is due in part to several factors. The original text was updated shortly prior to submission, and Springer did an outstanding production job of publishing the book quickly. The authorship of the atlas is broad based, with top international researchers in the field as contributors. Because the book is written by individuals involved in cutting-edge research, it includes information that has only subsequently appeared in the peer-reviewed literature. For example, computer-aided diagnosis is well covered in the atlas, even though commercialization of this software is not expected until next year. Thus, several topics are ahead of their time, thus keeping the contents relevant.

The nine chapters reprinted here represent the contribution of 16 experts in the field, and their subject matter helps readers understand current discussions about CT colonography. For instance, the chapter on accuracy is a useful reference when evaluating the recent publication of several clinical trials, particularly the screening trial by P.J. Pickhardt and coworkers, which stimulated strong interest in CTC by the general radiology community and the public. Some advances in CTC examination technique with automated insufflation, stool tagging, and electronic subtraction are also discussed in the book and have progressed further since then. Volume CT scanners capable of scanning 40 to 64 slices in one second are now available. Additional anticipated developments, including the commercialization of computer-aided detection of polyps and advances in CTC reading software promise to make CTC more accurate and easier to interpret in the near future. Insurance companies are gradually considering reimbursement, and CPT codes for virtual colonoscopy now exist. There is always a discrepancy between the examination performance and interpretation methods used in the peer-reviewed literature versus those that result when the exam is performed with state-of-the-art equipment and training. I anticipate that well-trained radiologists will outperform the accuracy reported in many clinical trials. This is in contrast to the normative assumption that experts in a research setting may achieve a higher sensitivity and positive predictive value in comparison to a busy clinical practice. I am confident that continued strides will be made in the immediate future to promote this technology in the marketplace and to improve the compliance of the public with colon cancer screening recommendations.

The gastroenterology community has largely accepted the fact that virtual colonoscopy, if interpreted by an experienced radiologist, is the best alternative to optical colonoscopy and can be used for patients who have an incomplete optical colonoscopy, usually on the same day. Many experts opine that screening virtual colonoscopy for average-risk patients will free-up a busy colonoscopy schedule to do more high-risk patients who are more likely to have an abnormal exam. Some gastroenterologists are even trying to learn how to interpret virtual colonoscopy themselves, leaving the extracolonic findings to the radiologist. I think that the emerging data on flat lesions in particular, covered by Dr. Jeff Fidler in Part II of the original atlas, underscore the importance of a careful 2D interpretation of images, even if a primary 3D read is used to search for polyps. This is one of many reasons why I believe that virtual colonoscopy should be the domain of the radiologist. Both radiologists and nonradiologists will find this "fundamentals" version an excellent way to learn about the issues and controversies.

Lastly, I would like to thank all the contributors, researchers, support staff and publication personnel who helped advance this technology and who contributed to the original version of the atlas as listed in the foreword. In the preparation of Part I of the atlas reprinted in the "fundamentals," I thank Marc Levine, MD, for reviewing the manuscript. I thank my publisher, Rob Albano and his staff at Springer, who worked with me on this project from concept to completion. Lastly and most dearly, I thank my wife Yisraela, our daughter Eliana, and my children Toby, Yitzchak, and Laya and to my wife's children Rachel, Shlomie and Yoni Marshall, for giving me the time and support needed to complete this task. The dedication page of the atlas as reprinted shows a dedication to my family and in memory of my father Albert Dachman, zl'. However, my mother Esther Deborah Dachman, zl', recently passed away and I rededicate this issue in her memory as well.

I hope that this issue of the atlas is as well received as was the initial version. I hope the audience of radiologists, gastroenterologists, practitioners, researchers, and residents find this atlas a valuable addition to the literature and enjoyable to read.

Chicago, Illinois   *Abraham H. Dachman, MD*

Contents

Preface   vii
Contributors   xi

1 Virtual Colonoscopy: The Inside Story   1
  David J. Vining

2 Background and Significance   4
  Seth N. Glick

3 How Accurate Is CT Colonography?   14
  Judy Yee and Elizabeth McFarland

4 How to Perform and Interpret a Virtual Colonoscopic Examination . . .   24
  Michael Macari and Abraham H. Dachman

5 Patient Preparation   47
  Michael Zalis

6 Advanced 3D Display Methods   53
  Christopher F. Beaulieu, David S. Paik, Sandy Napel,
  and R. Brooke Jeffrey, Jr.

7 MR Colonography   65
  Thomas C. Lauenstein and Jörg F. Debatin

8 Future Directions: Computer-Aided Diagnosis   79
  Ronald M. Summers and Hiroyuki Yoshida

9 A Word About Radiation Dose   90
  James A. Brink

Index 107

Contributors

Christopher F. Beaulieu, MD, PhD
Associate Professor of Radiology
Department of Radiology
Stanford University Medical Center
Stanford, CA 94305-5119, USA

James A. Brink, MD
Professor of Diagnostic Radiology
Vice-Chairman of Clinical Affairs
Department of Diagnostic Radiology
Yale University School of Medicine
New Haven, CT 06520, USA

Abraham H. Dachman, MD
Professor of Radiology
The University of Chicago Medical
  Center
Chicago, IL 60637-1470, USA

Jörg F. Debatin, MD, MBA
Department of Diagnostic Radiology
University Hospital Essen
Essen D-45122, Germany

Seth N. Glick, MD
Clinical Professor of Radiology
University of Pennsylvania Medical
  School
Presbyterian Medical Center
Philadelphia, PA 19104-4385, USA

R. Brooke Jeffrey, Jr., MD
Professor and Chief of Abdominal
  Imaging
Department of Radiology
Stanford University Medical Center
Stanford, CA 94305-5119, USA

Thomas C. Lauenstein, MD
Department of Diagnostic Radiology
University Hospital Essen
Essen D-45122, Germany

Michael Macari, MD
Assistant Professor of Radiology
NYU Medical Center
New York, NY 10016, USA

Elizabeth McFarland, MD
Associate Professor of Radiology
Mallinckrodt Institute of Radiology
St. Louis, MO 63130, USA

Sandy Napel, PhD
Associate Professor of Radiology
Department of Radiology
Stanford University Medical Center
Stanford, CA 94305-5119, USA

David S. Paik, PhD
Graduate Student
Department of Medical Informatics
Stanford University
Stanford, CA 94305-5119, USA

Ronald M. Summers, MD, PhD
Department of Radiology
National Institutes of Health
Bethesda, MD 20892, USA

David J. Vining, MD
Associate Professor
Department of Radiology
Wake Forest University Health
 Sciences Center
Winston-Salem, NC 27157, USA

Judy Yee, MD
Vice Chair of Radiology
University of California, San
 Francisco
Chief of Radiology
San Francisco Veterans Affairs
 Medical Center
San Francisco, CA 94121, USA

Hiroyuki Yoshida, PhD
Department of Radiology
The University of Chicago Medical
 Center
Chicago, IL 60637-1470, USA

Michael Zalis, MD
Instructor of Radiology
Harvard Medical School
Assistant Radiologist
Massachusetts General Hospital
Boston, MA 02114, USA

1

Virtual Colonoscopy: The Inside Story

David J. Vining

My inspiration for developing virtual colonoscopy (VC) was born of the marriage of two very different technologies—each significant in its own right but never before brought together. As a Winthrop fellow in Body Imaging/3D Imaging research at the Johns Hopkins Hospital from 1992 to 1993, I was exposed to many new and exciting technologies, including the introduction of spiral computed tomography (CT) scanning and the latest in virtual reality (VR) computer processing. It occurred to me early on that the computer technology I used to operate a flight simulator game on my home computer might also allow me to navigate the volume of data provided by spiral CT. In other words, combining these two technologies would enable me literally to travel inside the human body.

It was not until July 1993 that I began serious research into the development of VC. In my pursuit of an academic career, I interviewed with over half a dozen institutions, sharing with each department chairman my crazy idea to "fly inside the bowels." Only one individual took me seriously, however—C. Douglas Maynard, MD, Chairman of Radiology at the Bowman Gray School of Medicine of Wake Forest University.

When confronted with my request for expensive computer equipment, Dr. Maynard responded "No problem. Tell me what you need." I asked Dr. Maynard, "How about $25,000 to start?" and he quipped, "No problem!" I countered with "$50,000?" and "$75,000?" only to hear "No problem!" each time. Finally, I challenged him with "How about $250,000?" to which he said calmly, "That might be a problem, but I'll work on getting it for you."

When I arrived at Bowman Gray in summer 1993, Dr. Maynard had over $100,000 of equipment and software waiting for me in a dedicated research laboratory. He told me to "Go to work and do good things." Eventually, Dr. Maynard's original investment led to more than $5 million in research funding and more than a dozen US patents. His vision, generosity, and support made it possible for me to create and develop an entirely new segment of the health-care industry, now widely recognized as virtual endoscopy.

The essence of VC is simply to cleanse a patient's bowels, distend the colon with gas, scan the abdomen and pelvis with spiral CT, and use computers to construct a 3D virtual environment of the colon. The system allows a radiologist to fly through the colon to look for polyps and masses. One of my brave radiology colleagues, David Gelfand, MD, volunteered for the first "virtual colonoscopy" examination in September 1993. Dr. Gelfand underwent a standard bowel cleansing regimen and allowed me to insert a barium enema catheter into his rectum and insufflate his colon with room air using a hand-bulb insufflator. The spiral CT scan was performed on a General Electric HiSpeed Advantage Helical scanner that took approximately 50 seconds to complete with 5-mm collimation at 2:1 pitch.

The overall computer processing time required to generate the first VC fly-through took more than 8 hours to complete using a Silicon Graphics Crimson computer and Explorer software. Since then, there have been substantial improvements in several key technologies—a multislice helical CT scan now takes about 15 seconds to cover the abdomen and pelvis, and image analysis can be completed in approximately 10 minutes. However, in the early days there were many challenges such as the absence of the DICOM image standard required for proprietary CT images to be extracted from the scanner and transferred to the Silicon Graphics computer during a pain-staking operation. The computational power required to process the 250 Mb of CT data (500 images reconstructed at 1-mm intervals) was substantial for that time, so the data had to be divided into "colon segments" to perform segmental fly-throughs. Thankfully, technology has advanced a long way since then!

In February 1994, Dr. Gelfand and I presented the first VC fly-through video accompanied by the sounds of Wagner's "Ride of the Valkyries" at the annual meeting of the Society of Gastrointestinal Radiologists held in Maui. Needless to say, the audience was left with a lasting impression.

The next public VC presentation occurred at the National Cancer Institute's International Workshop on Colorectal Cancer Screening held in Bethesa, Md, in June 1994. This 3-day multidisiplinary conference covered all aspects of colorectal cancer research, prevention, diagnosis, and treatment. The gastroenterologists in attendance were having a great time bashing the radiologists' defense of the barium enema. When I introduced the VC concept at that meeting, I began my presentation with, "It's the bottom of the 9th inning, score is 3 to 0 in favor of the gastroenterologists, bases are loaded, and a new radiologist is up to bat." It was clear that the gastroenterology community, after seeing VC in action, realized that a new radiological procedure could impact the future of their practice.

Grants awarded from the North Carolina Baptist Hospital in 1993 and by the National Science Foundation in 1995 supported my continuing research in the field. Since those early days, researchers at Wake Forest University, as well as from around the world, have pursued improvements to the VC procedure, including the use of volume rendering, stool opacification and subtraction, electronic carbon dioxide insufflators, and computer-assisted diagnosis (CAD) of colon polyps. However, most practitioners of VC today agree that 2D review of CT images at a workstation is sufficient for lesion detection and that 3D imaging can be reserved for problem solving (e.g., determining if a suspicious finding represents a true polyp or merely a complex haustral fold).

The first commercial VC product to appear on the market was General Electric's Navigator, introduced at the Radiological Society of North America's annual meeting in November 1995. Today, more than 20 virtual endoscopy products are available.

Future Developments

Future challenges for VC are not necessarily technical in nature but related more to economics and public policy. Acceptance, pricing, reimbursement, and competing technologies are all major hurdles to be overcome. The public is enamored by this new VC procedure, but the medical community and public policy groups are more cautious with their support—convincing evidence from large-scale clinical trials comparing VC to conventional colonoscopy will be necessary to sway these groups in favor of VC. Affordable pricing for the VC procedure, especially to make it competitive against other available colon screening methods, will require consensus among radiology practices. Finally, it is important to recognize the fact that evolving technologies, such as stool screening for DNA markers, could also impact the value of VC as a screening tool. Nevertheless, VC is poised today to make an important contribution in the fight against colorectal cancer, the second-leading cancer killer in America.

2

Background and Significance

Seth N. Glick

Colorectal cancer is the second leading cause of cancer deaths. The mortality from this disease has improved slightly as a result of several factors, including earlier diagnosis, progress in therapeutic interventions, and, possibly, prevention. However, the impact has not been dramatic. The primary explanation is that our advances in knowledge and technology have not been implemented on a programmatic population basis. This deficiency has resulted from slow and insufficient dissemination of information to health-care professionals and the public, which has produced a relative lack of recognition and interest in this area. However, in the last decade there have been several developments that have catalyzed resurgence in awareness and action in understanding the potential benefit of colorectal cancer screening.

Historical Perspective on Colon Cancer Screening

In the mid-1970s, the concept of the adenoma–carcinoma sequence became popularized, primarily as a result of the research of Basil Morson (Day and Morson 1978). The basic principle is that there is an orderly and temporally consistent cytohistological and morphological progression from normal mucosa to advanced carcinoma. The initial lesion is the benign adenoma, which takes the form of a discrete mucosal elevation or polyp. Whereas small adenomatous polyps are common, with their prevalence increasing with age, a small percentage increase in size, resulting in histological alterations manifested by increased villous components and/or cytological deterioration described in degrees of cellular atypia or dysplasia. The critical size threshold was determined to be 1 cm because the frequency of more advanced changes in lesions above this size markedly increased. Further, there was a direct correlation between growth and the probability that the neoplasm contained malignant foci. This theory could not be directly proven and the evidence was circumstantial but the argument was convincing. The support came from several observations including the failure to identify small (<5 mm) pure carcinomas, as well as the combination of benign and malignant elements in adenomatous polyps with the frequency of associated cancer being size

4

related. Two other key corollaries to the adenoma–carcinoma sequence are that most colorectal cancers are derived through this pathway and that the time required for such progression is universally slow, on the order of 10 years or longer. The former was based upon the rarity of small carcinomas without benign components and the latter was extrapolated from demographic data where the age prevalence for carcinoma rises significantly approximately 10 years after the adenoma prevalence rate sharply increases. This model of colorectal carcinogenesis became generally accepted in the scientific community. Coincident with the dominance of this doctrine was the development of improved techniques for the detection and removal of adenomatous polyps. Reports on the high accuracy of the double-contrast barium enema in diagnosing colorectal polyps, in particular significant lesions larger than 1 cm were published (Glick 2000). Further, fiberoptic colonoscopy was shown to be sensitive for the identification of most polyps and proven to be a relatively safe procedure for the performance of polypectomy. However, these modalities were being utilized almost exclusively in symptomatic individuals whereby polyps were found and removed incidentally in the course of investigation for move advanced disease. Unfortunately, benign adenomas rarely cause symptoms. Given the level of consensus regarding the adenoma–carcinoma sequence, it would be intuitive to assume that, in theory, the removal of all adenomas in a timely manner should effectively prevent colorectal cancer and eliminate death from this disease. Nevertheless, there were no concentrated efforts to promote any form of screening in the asymptomatic population. This was related to lack of sufficient information on the epidemiology of the disease as well as prevailing issues pertaining to requisites for screening recommendations.

Existing screening proposals were predominantly centered on the detection of cancer, not polyps. Further, it was in general believed that most cancers (over 75%) arose in the distal colon within reach of the sigmoidoscope. Initially, screening consisted of a digital rectal examination and, possibly, a rigid sigmoidoscopy or stool testing for occult blood. Even the latter was performed inappropriately, being performed at the time of rectal examination rather than the current more systematic and rigorous process. With the addition of flexible sigmoidoscopy, the focus was predominantly on the left side of the colon. However, over the next 15 to 20 years a number of studies indicated that colorectal cancers (and adenomas) were more uniformly distributed throughout the colon. Even these relatively limited screening strategies were not widely adopted. A lack of appreciation and acceptance of the magnitude of an individual's risk and lack of confidence in the effectiveness of screening tests by both patient and primary caregivers were major factors. Reimbursement concerns, inconvenience, and the actual test experiences were certainly other factors. These all relate to issues at the patient–physician level. At the same time, policy makers for public health recommendations had specific requirements to be met before endorsing any form of screening. Unlike the case-finding dynamic that occurs in the usual practice of patient-generated health-care interaction, screening commits far greater financial and health-care resources. It also creates an environment in which there is the potential for psychological and physical morbidity from the screening process and subsequent interventions for individuals who are relatively well and the probability of disease-related benefit remains relatively low. Thus, the decision to advocate screening is dependent on proof that screening tests and follow-up treatment are effective in reducing morbidity and mortality from a major health-care burden and, in addition, meet defined standards of cost effectiveness. The latter is to ensure that limited financial resources would not be better utilized for other medical conditions. Thus, in essence, successful screening requires proof of effectiveness, advocacy by influential groups and providers, availability and access to screening tests, and acceptance by the target population. The last factor will be greatly affected by an individual's level of health-care motivation and the inconvenience and discomfort of undergoing a screening test.

Despite the acceptance of the adenoma–carcinoma sequence, convincing scientific evidence for screening effectiveness (i.e., that it reduces mortality) did not exist. As previously mentioned, the primary screening mechanism for the entire colon was the fecal occult blood test repeated at regular intervals, usually on an annual basis. As a test for detecting cancer, it is necessary to show that when cancer is found in asymptomatic individuals any apparent increase in length of survival is not due to earlier diagnosis (lead time bias) and any shift toward improved stages is not a function of finding indolent cancers (length time bias). Panels convened to assess screening procedures imposed strict criteria to determine the scientific quality of the studies necessary for the findings to be considered valid. The benchmark was the prospective, blinded, randomized, controlled trial. However, the retrospective case-control study was deemed a suitable alternative. In 1992, the first study supporting the effectiveness of colorectal screening was published (Selby et al. 1992). In this case-control study, it was found that individuals who had undergone rapid sigmoidoscopy had a reduced odds ratio for the probability of developing fatal cancer within the reach of the sigmoidoscope. There was no difference in screening exposure in those with fatal cancer proximally. It was unclear from the study details exactly how such screening produced its effect in the distal colon, as there were no cured cancers identified in the group without fatal rectal cancer. Subsequently, in 1993, a randomized trial demonstrated colorectal cancer mortality reduction through screening with fecal occult blood testing (Mandel et al. 1993). The presumed mechanism of action was a shift in the proportion of earlier-stage cancers and, in particular, a marked reduction in the percentage with metastatic disease at diagnosis. The first major panel to incorporate the findings of these studies was the US Preventative Services Task Force, which supported screening with either sigmoidoscopy or fecal occult blood testing. Combination strategies, although recommended by some groups, lacked evidence. In 1993, the findings of the multi-institutional National Polyp Study were published (Winawer et al. 1993). This study assessed the outcome after the surveillance of individuals who had had adenomatous polyps removed at entry. The observed cancer incidence was markedly reduced compared to three published reference groups. Although impressive, this still did not demonstrate mortality reduction. In 1994, a multidisciplinary panel of experts was convened by the Agency for Health Care Policy and Research

(AHCPR) to develop recommendations for colorectal cancer screening. There were five important conceptual innovations that resulted from their proceedings. The first was the relaxation of the stringent evidence-based criteria. Instead of directly linking a specific modality to the existing evidence for screening, it was accepted that if the early detection of cancer reduces mortality any procedure that reliably detects colon cancer could be assumed to be effective as well. This allowed for the second major change, the consideration of the double-contrast barium enema and colonoscopy for the general population. Integral to the proposal of such increasingly invasive and expensive procedures was the understanding that screening is not intended to be a one-time event but rather a long-term program of repeated application. If such tests are more thorough and can be performed at prolonged intervals, it minimizes their negative features. Thus, this panel became the first to incorporate decision analysis and modeling to assess the aggregate impact, both favorable and unfavorable, of several screening strategies. As part of this process, cost-effectiveness analysis was also included. It was determined in a study by the Office of Technology Assessment that all approaches being reviewed were most cost effective than accepted benchmarks for other medical interventions. The fourth significant advance was the refinement of the understanding of cancer risk categories, adding a group termed "above average risk" to the traditional stratification of high and low risk. Decisions regarding whom to screen, how to screen, and how often to screen tend to be based on a complex integration of the magnitude of risk, the natural history of the disease, and the diverse characteristics of the screening test(s). Historically, any form of screening, especially with more aggressive strategies, had been reserved for high-risk groups to make exposure and resource utilization more efficient. However, it was also appreciated that a high preponderance of the overall tumor burden came from those at average or above average risk. The latter category included those with a previous history of cancer or large adenoma (especially with more advanced pathology) and those with a first-degree family history with the relative being under age 55 at diagnosis. Recog-nizing that risk represented a gradual continuum based on age and other individual variables, the screening recommendations that were proposed did not differ dramatically but blended in a tailored overlapping manner based upon the level of risk. Thus, the fifth and most significant product of the panel was the development of recommendations that included *a menu of screening options* based upon the knowledge that all the screening strategies should work to varying degrees and overall participation in screening could be augmented by enhancing availability and the potential for compliance. Inherent in this dynamic would be the necessity for informed shared decision making by the health-care givers and the target population. Further, choice would be based on the relative trade-offs of the differing approaches. Those guidelines were published in 1997 (Table 2.1) (Winawer et al. 1997). Closely following, and to some degree influenced by, the AHCPR guidelines were colorectal cancer screening recommendations put forth by the American Cancer Society that were almost identical (Byers et al. 1997). Also, opportunistically synchronized with these policy documents were successful legislative ini-

TABLE 2.1. 1997 American Cancer Society screening guidelines for colorectal cancer.

Average-risk patients
  Asymptomatic, > age 50
    Initial exam
      1. Fecal occult blood test (FOBT) and flexible sigmoidoscopy with digital rectal exam (DRE)
      or
      2. Total colon examination (TCE) with DRE (colonoscopy or double-contrast barium enema [DCBE])
    Follow-up
      1. FOBT q y, flexible sigmoidoscopy q 5 y
      or
      2. Colonoscopy q 10 y or DCBE q 5–10 y
Moderate-risk patients
  Single small polyp
    Initial exam   Colonoscopy
    Follow-up   TCE within 3 y from polypectomy; *if normal*, return to average-risk guidelines
  Large polyp or multiple small polyps
    Initial exam   Colonoscopy
    Follow-up   TCE within 3 y from polypectomy; *if normal*, TCE q 5 y
  Post-CRC resection
    Initial exam   TCE within 1 y
    Follow-up   TCE in 3 y; *if normal*, TCE q 5 y
  CRC or adenomatous polyps in first-degree relative
    Initial exam   TCE at age 40
                          or
                          10 y prior to family case
    Follow-up   TCE q 5 y
High-risk patients
  Familial adenomatous polyposis
    Initial exam   Endoscopy at puberty; counseling, genetic testing
    Follow-up   If genetics +, colectomy; otherwise, endoscopy q 1–2 y
  Hereditary nonpolyposis colorectal cancer
    Initial exam   Colonoscopy and counseling at age 21
    Follow-up   Colonoscopy q 2y until age 40, then q 1 y
  Inflammatory bowel disease
    Initial exam   Colonoscopy with biopsy 8 y after start of colitis
    Follow-up   Colonoscopy every 1–2 y

Source: Adapted with permission from Byers et al. (1997).

tiatives through which Medicare began providing coverage for the proposed screening modalities. The reimbursements did not include colonoscopy for those at average risk but this coverage was added in 2001.

Since 1997, awareness of and participation in colorectal cancer screening has increased somewhat but not to the levels desired and certainly not approaching that of breast cancer screening. Enhanced media attention to screening through reports on the subject as well as transmission of the findings of new studies has provided greater visibility and interest. The National Colorectal Cancer Roundtable—a consortium of medical societies, advocacy groups, government-sponsored organizations, and motivated individuals—was formed for the purpose of promoting awareness and involvement in screening. Research projects have been ongoing in multiple areas to improve compliance, provide a better understanding of the potential implications of the various screening strategies, and increase the knowledge base concerning the epidemiology and genesis of this disease.

Current Screening Practices

There currently are several proposed screening choices, including fecal occult blood testing, flexible sigmoidoscopy, a combination of the two, double-contrast barium enema, and colonoscopy. As mentioned, none of these choices are ideal and all have strengths and limitations. Without going into great detail, the fecal occult blood test is inexpensive and readily applied at the mass level. However, it is insensitive to adenomatous polyps and a single application has only fair sensitivity for colorectal cancer, necessitating strict adherence to repeat testing. Flexible sigmoidoscopy visualizes less than half of the bowel but a protocol of performing colonoscopy after an adenoma is detected improves the yield to approximately 75% of the significant neoplasms. Although it is much safer and less expensive than colonoscopy and does not require sedation, such a program will overlook a significant portion of lesions because of their location in the proximal colon. Although, in theory, the addition of annual fecal occult blood testing should partially compensate for this limitation, there is no evidence if, or to what degree, the benefits are additive. Further, any improvement is directed toward early cancer detection rather than disease prevention.

Colonoscopy is the definitive procedure for evaluating the colon and can be both diagnostic and therapeutic. Although the risks of perforation and hemorrhage are relatively low, they are much higher than with any of the screening alternatives. Unlike sigmoidoscopy, colonoscopy also requires more intensive preparation, which many find unpleasant. The completion rate for colonoscopy may vary from 75% to 99% depending on the examiner's skills, anatomic variations, prior abdominal surgery, and the patient's reaction to the anesthesia. In either endoscopic scenario, whether sigmoidoscopy or colonoscopy, there may be a significant number of individuals who are averse to having a tube placed in their bowel and they are apprehensive regarding the discomfort they may experience. The double-contrast barium enema is relatively inexpensive (equivalent to sigmoidoscopy) and is the safest of all the structural screening tests. However, thorough colonic preparation is a requirement and the test itself, while usually associated with minimal to mild discomfort, may be perceived as being painful. A preponderance of literature consisting of observational studies suggests that this test can detect 80% to 90% of the large adenomas and 85% to 95% of cancers (Glick 2000). However, a randomized controlled trial comparing double-contrast barium enema to colonoscopy reported a detection rate of only half the large adenomas (Glick 2000). While this is only a single study and there are a number of limitations regarding the generalizability of the findings, this study has been used to advocate colonoscopy over the double-contrast barium enema. Another important factor in the decline of the barium enema is the waning interest of radiologists in performing this procedure. The low reimbursement of the barium enema in conjunction with its labor-intensive nature has also been a deterrent. In addition, radiologists' skills have greatly deteriorated due to the decreased number of studies performed as a result of increased utilization of colonoscopy. This has impacted on practicing radiologists as well as residents in training. Further, resident enthusiasm has gravitated toward more complex technology such as magnetic resonance imaging (MRI) and computed tomography (CT).

CT Colonography and Colon Cancer Screening

It is in this context that CT colonography (CTC) has emerged. The trend in colonic evaluation, in particular for screening, has shifted to total colonic evaluation. What currently exists for this purpose are two types of examinations. Colonoscopy is the definitive procedure but is associated with the greatest number of complications and expense, and there are questions about acceptability and availability to the masses at risk. The double-contrast barium enema, while having great potential and closely in accordance with traditional criteria for screening, is lacking because of the diminished skills and interest of radiologists and decreasing credibility due to opinions regarding its accuracy. Perceptions regarding the patient experience have also contributed to its markedly decreased utilization. The question then arises as to how CTC can overcome the respective limitations of these two modalities. Its potential must also be viewed in terms of alternative techniques that are currently being developed, such as stool evaluation for genetic mutations. Much is unknown regarding CTC and it is difficult to perform a comparative analysis at present. There are a number of issues that need to be resolved. Several of these are interrelated and impact upon each other. First is its accuracy for cancer and large adenomas in conjunction with the prevailing practice for the management of small polyps. Most studies concerning accuracy have been performed in highly controlled settings and under these conditions have produced results approaching that of colonoscopy for larger and more significant lesions (Fenlon et al. 1999). If this can be consistently reproduced in the general population, then CTC should have tremendous impact. Although the reimbursement for CTC has yet to be established, it would be expected to be somewhere between the amount for colonoscopy and double-contrast barium enema. Given the prevalence of small polyps and the dubious benefit from their removal, if a high percentage of CTC studies lead to colonoscopy the net costs may be prohibitive. However, if a protocol could be established whereby such polyps were to be ignored (e.g., age dependent) or followed with CT at a reasonably prolonged interval then the financial limitations of CT as a screening test would become diminished. Other issues that are tangential but have both economic and medical repercussions include the importance of radiation exposure and the consequences (both positive and negative) of the discovery of findings unrelated to the colon.

The second key variable is the willingness of the general public to undergo CT colonography as opposed to other screening options or, more importantly, no form of screening whatsoever. CTC, like colonoscopy and double-contrast barium enema, requires both an uncomfortable preprocedural preparation and intraprocedural distension of the colon by gas. Unlike colonoscopy, there is no need for sedation, which may be viewed favorably by some and negatively by others. However, most attractive is that the overall time required during which an individual undergoes the actual intervention is extremely short, which should make it a better experience. Further, research is currently taking place that would eliminate the need for colonic cleansing (i.e., "prepless"). This would certainly enhance compliance but it must be proven that the sensitivity and specificity are maintained.

A third area of concern is that the inherent nature of the technique requires the review of an extremely large number of images. This can occupy a significant amount of a radiologist's time if proper scrutiny is to be applied. Failure to be properly diligent could be detrimental to performance. Such dedication could be limited by the volume of other studies that exist in a busy radiology practice. The current review time for experienced radiologists is reported to be approximately 5 to 20 minutes per case but can be much longer. Further, there could be a fatigue factor that limits the numbers of studies that can be performed. However, another area of investigation that offers promise in overcoming these problems is computer-assisted diagnosis. This application could, if perfected, offer the radiologist the ability to focus on a few regions that may contain significant lesions without necessarily evaluating every image. [Editor's note: Also, novel software programs such as "virtual pathology" may not only reduce interpretation time but also the level of expertise needed to properly interpret the examination].

Obstructing Cancer and Incomplete Colonoscopy

CTC has already achieved a role in the evaluation of patients with incomplete colonoscopy. The patient who is already prepared and has undergone an incomplete colonoscopy can be accommodated for a same-day, unscheduled CTC examination, thus obviating the need for a return visit and repeat preparation. Morrin et al. (2000) studied 40 patients with CT within 2 hours of an incomplete colonoscopy and, showing the portion of the colon that was not visualized by endoscopy in over 90% of patients, found a probable cause for the obstruction in 74% of patients. Further, patients preferred CT over colonoscopy. Fenlon showed that CT depicted all 29 occlusive carcinomas and also fully evaluated the proximal colon in 26 of 29 patients. CT also demonstrated two synchronous cancers and 24 polyps in the proximal colon, many of which were subsequently confirmed by endoscopy, although none could be palpated at surgery. Identification of the synchronous cancers in two patients altered the surgical plan. CT was also more accurate than colonoscopy in localizing the cancers, which may be helpful in preoperative planning.

Royster et al. (1997) reported a 100% sensitivity in detecting masses ≥2 cm on CTC. Several investigators have shown the utility and effectiveness of virtual colonoscopy to image the colon proximal to obstructing lesions. Macari et al. (1999) reported on 20 patients with incomplete colonoscopy, 10 of whom had barium enema. Two lesions were found by CT in the portion of the colon not seen by colonoscopy and confirmed by barium enema and the other eight were normal on both examinations.

Extracolonic Findings

Ironically, the incidence of extracolonic findings seems to be potentially as important as detection of colonic polyps (Dachman, 2002). This analysis is in particular interesting in light of recent heated debate regarding use of CT as a general head-to-toe screening tool. Dachman reported 26 incidental findings in 44 patients, only 1 of which (3-cm adrenal mass) resulted in additional work-up (Glick 2000). Other findings included four patients with hepatic steatosis, four with gallstones, and one with an inguinal hernia. In a group of 40 patients with incomplete colonoscopy, Morrin found a 13% incidence of significant extracolonic findings, such as aortic aneurysm, complex ovarian cyst, partially obstructing ventral hernia, and large fibroid uterus with bowel compression. Hopper found potentially significant extracolonic findings in 10% (10/100) of patients and insignificant extracolonic findings in an additional 80%. Significant findings included spinal block, 4-cm adrenal mass, questionable abscess around the femoral neck, 4-cm aortic aneurysm, porcelain gallbladder, large herniated disc with edematous nerve root, narrow-neck ventral abdominal wall hernia containing colon, fractured orthopedic hardware with a lumbar subluxation, and severe bladder wall thickening in a woman. Hara formally studied 264 consecutive virtual colonoscopy examinations using two observers and found that 11% (30/264) had highly important extracolonic findings that resulted in further examination in 7% (18) of patients. Six patients underwent surgery because of these findings. Two patients with findings of moderate or low importance underwent additional imaging. They also did a cost analysis and found that evaluation of important extracolonic findings can help detect serious disease with little additional cost. These findings may be as important as the finding of polyps in these patients and deserve further study.

Conclusion

It is clear that CTC is a rapidly developing technology that has the potential to make a major contribution for decreasing the morbidity and mortality from colorectal cancer. Exactly where it will interface and its actual future impact remain to be determined. However, it can be conservatively stated that a majority of the population do not undergo screening. If those who do not currently comply because of apprehension regarding existing modalities or because of limited access to colonoscopy, the existence of an alternative that is effective, accessible, and appealing to many of these individuals can be of considerable benefit to the aggregate public health.

3

How Accurate Is CT Colonography?

Judy Yee and Elizabeth McFarland

Computed tomography (CT) colonography (CTC), also referred to as virtual colonoscopy, has received widespread attention as a new tool for the noninvasive detection of colorectal polyps and cancer. Since the introduction of CTC in 1994, multiple preliminary studies have been performed to evaluate the sensitivity and specificity of CTC in different patient cohorts. During this time, there have been tremendous advances in the image acquisition and display capabilities of this evolving technology. Our purpose will be to first discuss specific parameters that may affect the performance results, followed by a review of studies performed to date.

Study Parameters

Patient Selection

Most of the published studies evaluating the accuracy of CTC have been performed in high-risk patients. These cohorts include patients with a personal or family history of colorectal cancer, patients with symptoms (iron-deficiency anemia, heme-positive stools, or hematochezia), or patients with prior polyps being followed for surveillance. The sensitivity and specificity of CTC for lesion detection in such polyp-rich patient populations may be higher than that in a screening population. Early studies evaluated well-characterized cohorts during the evolution of the technology, but these results cannot be extrapolated to a screening population. Future studies of test performance need to be performed in screening and surveillance populations in which disease prevalence is in general low.

Bowel Cleansing and Distention

Prior to the acquisition of CT data, patients are required to undergo a bowel cleansing regimen. Polyethylene glycol electrolyte lavage solution is the preferred agent by some gastroenterologists for bowel cleansing prior to colonoscopy. Polyethylene glycol is ingested in large volumes and is effective at cleansing the bowel. However, it often leaves excess residual fluid in the colon; therefore, it is known as a "wet prep." Residual fluid will obscure colonic lesions and lead to an increase in false negatives. The results from almost all published studies evaluating the performance of CTC for lesion detection are based on patients who have received polyethylene glycol solution as the colonic cleansing agent. Highly osmotic agents such as sodium phosphate (phosphosoda) and magnesium citrate tend to leave the colon relatively dry. However, these "dry preps" tend to leave more solid stool, which can lead to an increased number of false positives and false negatives.

Bowel distention is achieved by retrograde insufflation of the colon with either atmospheric air or carbon dioxide. Carbon dioxide has a steep diffusion gradient across the colonic wall and is resorbed much more rapidly than room air. It is thought to decrease patient discomfort, but it is not clear whether there is any significant effect on colonic distention or polyp detection. Preliminary findings of a prospective randomized study comparing manual insufflation of air vs carbon dioxide revealed similar distention and patient preference for the two gases (McDermott et al. 2001).

The use of glucagon as an antispasmodic agent has been controversial. There is evidence that glucagon does not have any significant effect in improving colonic distention or lesion detection for CTC (Yee et al. 1999; Morrin et al. 1999). Other reasons why glucagon is not likely to be used on a routine basis for CTC include cost issues and the faster acquisition times of multidetector CT scanners. Some of the more recent studies include patients who have not received glucagon.

CT Data Acquisition Protocol

Most of the published trials evaluating the diagnostic accuracy of CTC have been performed using a single-detector helical scanner. Single-detector CT protocols that have been studied include various collimations of 3, 5, and >5 mm. Trials are currently in progress exploring the potential for increased sensitivity and specificity using multidetector row CT. Thinner slices of 1- to 2-mm detector width may allow improved spatial resolution and increased sensitivity, in particular for smaller polyps and flat lesions. In addition, narrower collimation may allow easier distinction between polyps and residual stool. However, a higher sensitivity for polyp detection must not be offset by a lower specificity. Limitations of the use of thinner collimation include an increase in image noise that may compromise image quality, an increase in radiation dose to the patient, and larger data management demands.

Essentially all published studies evaluating the ability of CTC to detect polyps have used two-position scanning with supine and prone views. The use of scanning in opposing views has been found to improve colonic distention as well as polyp detection because of shifting of residual material that allows increased surface area visualization (Fletcher et al. 2000; Chen et al. 1999).

Image Display

The typical image displays used for CTC to date include the 2D multiplanar re-formations (2D MPR) and 3D endoluminal views. The 2D MPR allows a seam-less interactivity of axial, coronal, and sagittal planes for detection of focal in-traluminal lesions in a time-efficient manner (Fig 3.1). Other benefits include improved orientation from the extraluminal point of view and ability to evaluate the source attenuation data for improved characterization. The 3D endoscopic views provide an intraluminal visualization of the colonic mucosal surface (Figs 3.2 and 3.3). The 3D views can exploit different features, such as shaded-surface display or volume-rendered algorithms, color or monochromatic visual-ization, perspective lighting (to differentiate near field from far field), and man-ual or automated flight paths for navigation (Rubin et al. 1996; McFarland et al. 1997). Currently, most readers have used the time-efficient protocol of primary interpretation using the 2D MPR images, with selective correlation of focal find-ings with the 3D endoluminal images (Dachman et al. 1998; Macari et al. 2000). Further evaluations with 3D visualization as a primary method of evaluation need to be investigated as these capabilities evolve.

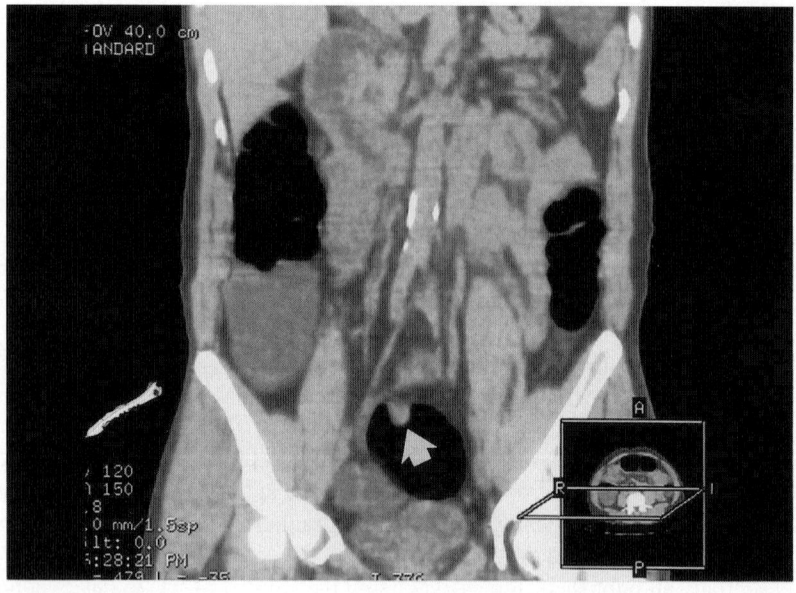

A

FIGURE 3.1. (**A**) Coronal reformatted view demonstrates a large sigmoid polyp (arrow). Differentiation from a thickened fold can be made by scrolling through the lesion on the 2D views.

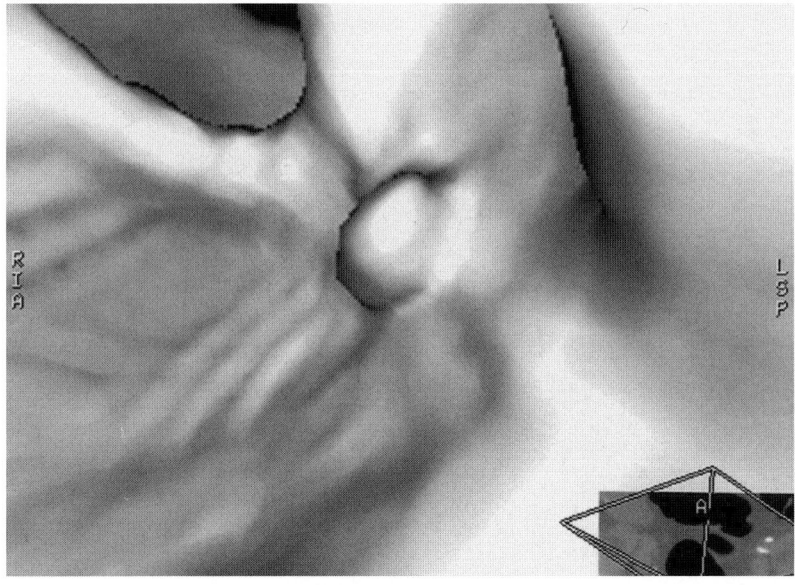

B

FIGURE 3.1. (*Continued*) (**B**) 3D endoscopic view shows the same polyp appearing as a focal protrusion into the lumen of the colon.

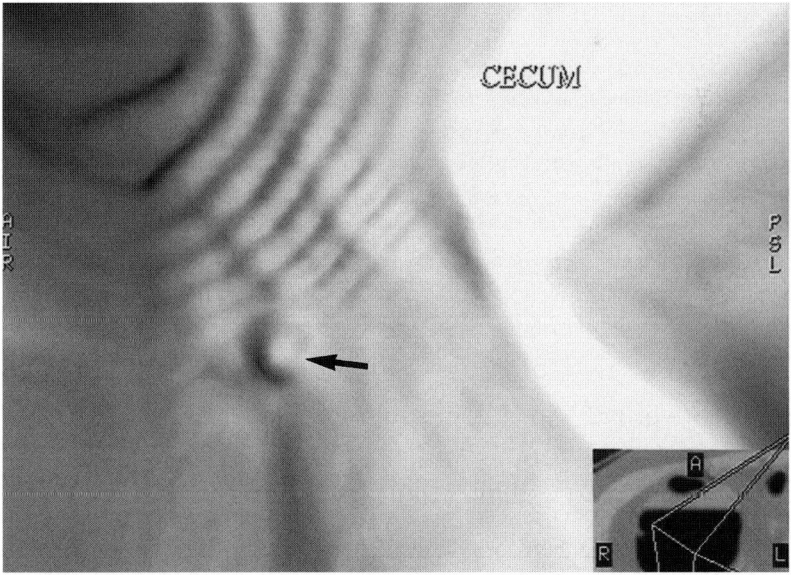

FIGURE 3.2. Excellent distention of the cecum allows detection of a small polyp (arrow) on the 3D endoluminal view.

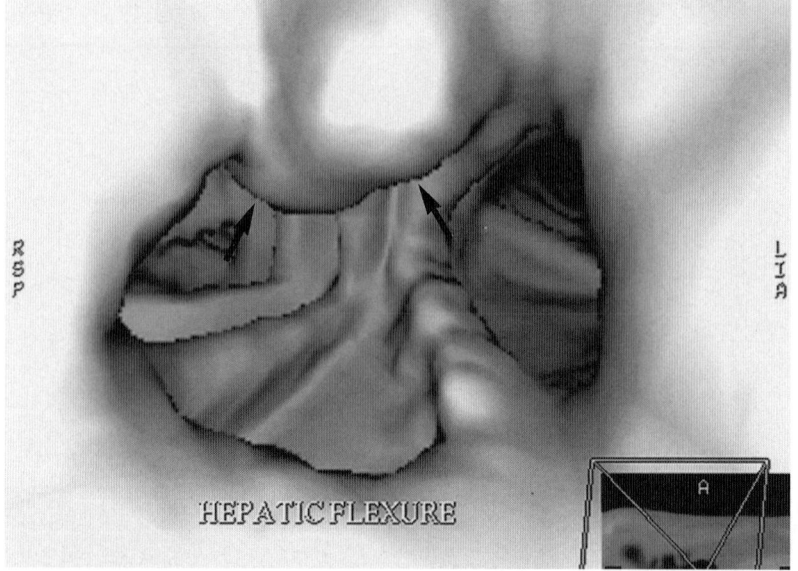

FIGURE 3.3. 3D endoscopic view demonstrates a large mass (arrows) in the hepatic flexure along the nondependent wall. A small amount of fluid is seen layering along the dependent wall.

Readers

To date, experienced abdominal radiologists have predominantly evaluated the early diagnostic performance of CTC. Many of the published studies have utilized single expert readers or consensus readings. Assessment of intra-and interobserver agreement is currently being performed (Pescatore et al. 2000; McFarland et al. 2000, 2002). The work of the American College of Radiology Imaging Network (ACRIN) represents the first large-scale multi-institutional efforts to evaluate newly trained and experienced readers. Future evaluations will require specific training protocols to familiarize new readers with different image display techniques and various sizes and morphologies of colorectal lesions.

Current Results Using 2D and Complete 3D

Yee et al. (2001) performed the largest single-center study to date evaluating CTC performance in 300 patients (Table 3.1). Approximately one-third of these patients were asymptomatic. Single-detector CT was used with 3-mm collimation, 1.5 to 2.0 pitch, 120 to 150 mA, and 1.5-mm reconstructions. Reader protocol consisted of complete interpretation of axial, reformatted, and endoluminal images in supine and prone positions. Interpretation was performed by two readers who evaluated 2D and 3D surface-rendered images in all patients, and a con-

TABLE 3.1. Performance data using complete 2D and 3D interpretation.

Study	CT type, collimation, SR vs VR	# Patients and type	By polyp sensitivity ≥10 mm	By polyp sensitivity 5–10 mm	By patient sensitivity ≥10 mm	By patient specificity ≥10 mm
Yee et al. 2001	SD, 3.0, SR	300 (204 high risk)	90.2%	80%	100%	—
Spinzi et al. 2001	SD, 5.0, SR	96 high risk	62%	56%	—	100%
Pescatore et al. 2000	SD, 5.0, SR	50 high risk	—	—	(<10 mm) 38%–63%	74%
Fenlon et al. 1999	SD, 5.0, VR	100 high risk	91%	82%	96%	96%
Royster et al. 1997	SD, 5.0, VR	20 + masses	100%	90%	100%	—

sensus reading was obtained. CTC had a 100% (8/8) sensitivity for the detection of carcinoma. Excellent results were also obtained using two different matching algorithms for larger polyps. Using direct by-polyp matching the sensitivity for polyp detection was 90.2% (74/82) for polyps 10 mm or larger and 80.1% (113/141) for polyps between 5 to 9.9 mm: Using the by-patient comparison, 100% (49/49) of patients with polyps measuring 10 mm or larger were identified and 93% (50/54) of patients with polyps measuring between 5 to 9.9 mm were identified on CTC. The positive-predictive value (PPV) and negative-predictive value (NPV) for clinically significant polyps measuring ≥10 mm was 80.8% and 97.2%, respectively.

Spinzi et al. (2001) obtained lower sensitivity results for the detection of polyps in a study of 96 high-risk or symptomatic patients. CTC was performed using 5-mm collimation, 2 pitch, 230 to 260 mA, and 2.5-mm reconstructions. 2D and complete 3D surface-rendered evaluation was performed by one radiologist. Per-polyp sensitivity for 10-mm or larger lesions was 62% (8/13) with a specificity of 100%. There was also low per-polyp sensitivity of 56% (18/32) for polyps smaller than 10 mm. This study found that CTC had a sensitivity of 88% (7/8) for the detection of cancers.

Fenlon et al. (1999) compared CTC and standard colonoscopy for polyp detection in 100 patients at high risk for colorectal neoplasia. The CT protocol consisted of 5-mm collimation, 1.25 pitch, 110 mA, and 2-mm reconstructions. 2D and complete 3D volume-rendered evaluation was performed by two radiologists who reviewed the CT studies jointly and arrived at a consensus reading. The per-polyp sensitivity of CTC was 91% (20/22) for polyps 10 mm or larger and 82% (33/40) for polyps 6 to 9 mm. Per-patient sensitivity and specificity as well as

PPV and NPV were all 96% for polyps 10 mm or larger. For polyps between 6 to 9 mm, per-patient sensitivity, specificity, PPV, and NPV were 94%, 92%, 92%, and 94%, respectively. Sensitivity results from this study are similar to the study by Yee et al. (2001).

Royster et al. (1997) performed a study evaluating 20 patients with known colonic masses found on fiberoptic colonoscopy. CTC was performed using 5-mm collimation, 1.25 pitch, 110 mA, and 2-mm reconstructions. 2D and complete 3D volume-rendered images were evaluated by two radiologists with a consensus reading obtained. All 20 masses measuring 20 mm or larger were identified. Per-polyp sensitivity for lesions measuring 10 mm or larger and for those between 6 and 10 mm were 100% (2/2) and 90% (9/10), respectively.

Current Results Using 2D with 3D for Problem Solving

Hara et al. (2001) compared single-detector vs multirow-detector CT for lesion detection in 237 patients. Seventy-seven patients underwent single-detector CTC with 5-mm collimation, 1.3 pitch, 70 mA, and 3-mm reconstructions. Using this protocol, three to four CT volumes were obtained with 3-cm overlap. The majority of patients (160) underwent multidetector CT scanning with 5-mm collimation, 0.75 pitch, 50 mA, and 3-mm reconstructions performed in one breath hold. Two of three radiologists who interpreted each of the studies used magnified axial images for the primary interpretation with 3D volume-rendered views for problem solving. CT results were considered positive if either of the two radiologists reported a finding. Per-polyp sensitivity for lesions larger than 10 mm was 89% (8/9) for single-detector CT vs 80% (8/10) for multidetector CT, with differences not found to be statistically significant. Per-patient sensitivity and specificity were 100% (5/5) and 90% (65/72) for single-detector CT vs 78% (7/9) and 93% (140/151) for multidetector CT, respectively, with differences also not found to be statistically significant. Although performance of CTC for polyp detection was similar for both single- and multidetector CT, it was found that colonic distention was better using multidetector CT with fewer respiratory artifacts.

In a study of 44 high-risk patients by Dachman et al. (1998), 2D images were used for primary interpretation and surface-rendered endoluminal views were reviewed only when needed to differentiate polyps from folds. Two radiologists interpreted each CT study independently. The CTC protocol consisted of 5-mm collimation, 1.5 pitch, 100 mA, and 2.5-mm reconstructions. A per-polyp sensitivity of 83% (5/6) was obtained for both readers for lesions 8 mm or larger with a specificity of 100%. The sensitivity for 5- to 8-mm polyps was 33% (1/3) for both readers. The endoluminal view was used for problem solving in 52% (23/44) of patients by both observers and did not significantly impact on interpretation times.

Morrin et al. (2000) evaluated 33 high-risk patients who did not receive intravenous contrast material and used a similar interpretation method in which surface-rendered endoluminal views were generated only in questionable areas found on the 2D views. CTC was performed using single- and multidetector scanners. Single-detector CT was performed on the majority of patients, and the protocol consisted of 3.0-mm collimation, 2 pitch, 120 mA, and 1.5-mm reconstructions. Multidetector CT protocol consisted of 2.5- to 5.0-mm slice thickness, 11.25- to 15-mm/s table speed, 200 mA in high-speed mode. Per-polyp sensitivity for 10- to 19-mm polyps and 5- to 9-mm polyps was 91% (11/12) and 58% (7/12), respectively. Per-patient sensitivity and specificity for the 10- to 19-mm polyps was 86% and 100%, respectively.

Fletcher et al. (2000) evaluated 180 patients with polyps or risk factors for colorectal cancer. Single-detector CT scanning was performed using 5-mm collimation, 70 mA, 1.3 pitch, and a 3-mm reconstruction interval. Three or four 20-second breath holds were required to cover the abdomen and pelvis with 3-cm overlap used to cover gaps. In addition, 89 patients were randomly assigned to receive oral iodinated contrast with a bowel-cleansing regimen the day before the CT. One reader interpreted the supine images alone and another reader evaluated both supine and prone data sets. Per-polyp sensitivity for lesions 10 mm or larger and for polyps between 5 and 9 mm were 75.2% (91/121) and 47.2% (67/142) respectively. Per-patient sensitivity and specificity for 10-mm or larger polyps were 85.4% and 93% respectively. It was found that the use of both supine and prone data sets significantly improved the ability to detect patients with polyps 5 mm or larger. The use of oral iodinated contrast in this study did not appear to improve polyp detection.

Macari et al. (2002) published a low-dose multidetector CT study in 105 high-risk patients. Images were acquired at 1-mm detector width, effective mAs of 50, and variable pitch to cover the abdomen and pelvis in 30 seconds. One reader evaluated the images with primary use of axial 2D as the major image display, with a mean interpretation time of 12 minutes. Sensitivity was 70% (19/27) for 6- to 9-mm lesions and 93% (13/14) for 10-mm and greater lesions. Overall specificity was found to be 98% (see Table 3.2).

TABLE 3.2. Performance data using 2D and 3D interpretation for problem solving.

Study	CT type, collimation, SR vs VR	# Patients and type	By polyp sensitivity ≥10 mm	By polyp sensitivity 5–10 mm	By patient sensitivity ≥10 mm	By patient specificity ≥10 mm
Macari et al. 2002	MD, 1.0, VR	105 high risk	92.9%	70.4%		97.7%
Hara et al. 2001	SD + MD 5.0, VR	237 high risk	80%–89%	—	78%–100%	90%–93%
Dachman et al. 1998	SD 5.0, SR	44 high risk	83% (>8 mm)	33%	83%	100%
Morrin et al. 2000	SD + MD 3.0, SR	33 high risk	91%	58%	86%	100%
Fletcher et al. 2000	SD 5.0, VR	180 high risk	75.2%	47.2%	85.4%	93%

Interobserver Agreement

Pescatore et al. (2000) performed a prospective study of 50 high-risk patients. CTC was performed in the supine position using 5-mm collimation, 1.5 pitch, 200 mA, and 2.5-mm reconstructions. 2D and complete 3D surface-rendered evaluation was performed by two investigator teams consisting of a radiologist and a gastroenterologist. Each team read out the first 24 patients, followed by evaluation of results. Then, each team read out the remaining patients. Per-patient sensitivity for 10-mm or larger polyps was 38% and 63% for teams 1 and 2, respectively, and specificity was 74% for both teams. The lower sensitivity results could be explained by many patients with poor preparation, scanning in only the supine position, suboptimal resolution of the software employed, and reader inexperience.

McFarland et al. (2000) initially evaluated inter- and intraobserver agreement in a retrospective library of 30 colonic segments containing 22 lesions using three different image display techniques. Images were acquired using single-detector CT, at 5-mm collimation, 8-mm table increment, and 2-mm reconstruction interval. Three experienced abdominal radiologists, who were recently trained with a teaching set of CTC cases, independently evaluated each case at two different testing periods. Results were similar between 2D MPR, thick-slab 3D MPR, and 3D perspective volume-rendered image display techniques. Sensitivity ranged from 77% to 86% for all polyps and 91% to 100% for polyps $\geq$10 mm (n = 11). Overall, intraobserver agreement was good for the three display techniques (κ = 0.6 to 1.0); however, interobserver agreement of 2D MPR was lower (κ = 0.53 to 0.80).

McFarland et al. (2002) also evaluated prospectively a polyp-rich cohort of 70 patients, using single detector CT (5-mm collimation, 8-mm table increment, 2-mm reconstruction interval). Four experienced abdominal radiologists independently evaluated each case using 2D MPR as the primary image display, with 3D volume rendered views to further characterize each finding. Analysis by polyp demonstrated a pooled sensitivity of 68% (range 60% to 78%) to detect 10 mm polyps (n = 40 polyps). Analysis by patient demonstrated a pooled sensitivity of 88% (range 82% to 89%) to detect patients with 10 mm and greater polyps (n = 28 patients). When sensitivity and area under the curve were analyzed by polyp size threshold, results among readers peaked at polyp diameters of approximately 10 mm. Interobserver agreement was 79% for all patients, 72% for patients with 6–9 mm polyps (n = 20) and 94% for patients with 10 mm and greater polyps (n = 28). When sensitivity and area under the curve were analyzed by polyp size threshold, results among readers peaked at polyp diameters of approximately 10 mm. Interobserver agreement was 79% for all patients, 72% for patients with6- to 9-mm polyps (n = 20) and 94% for patients with 10-mm or greater polyps (n = 28).

Future Areas of Validation

Future efforts to validate CTC will be challenged by the continued advances in CT acquisition and image processing capabilities. Optimization and standardization of the CT protocol will be necessary before further dissemination. Further evaluation of computed-aided diagnosis (Summers 2002), novel 3D image display techniques (Beaulieu et al. 1999; Reed and Johnson 1998), and stool tagging and subtraction (Zalis and Hahn 2001; Callstrom et al. 2001) will be needed. The diagnostic performance of CTC using a broader range of cases in community environments with less expert readers following a training period must be evaluated. Determination of what size lesion is considered "clinically significant" will be important (Glick 2000; Read et al. 1997; Rex and Cummings 1993). Multidisciplinary collaboration will be necessary for establishing screening and surveillance algorithms that account for important covariables, such as age, risk, and comorbidity. Comparison of the diagnostic performance of CTC to exisiting modalities such as flexible sigmoidoscopy, barium enema, and colonoscopy is also needed. In this way, the role of CTC as a part of the imaging armamentarium for colorectal cancer can be determined.

4

How to Perform and Interpret a Virtual Colonoscopic Examination

Michael Macari and Abraham H. Dachman

In this chapter, we discuss computed tomography (CT) of the cleansed colon performed in a manner to detect polyps and masses. The use of CT colonography (CTC) in the partially prepared or unprepared colon is discussed in chapter 5.

Technical considerations critical to the successful performance and interpretation of CTC are reviewed. This chapter presents an overview of how to perform and interpret an examination and will touch on some of the controversies.

Patient Preparation and Data Acquisition

Accepted principles regarding acceptable CTC technique include adequate colonic cleansing, maximal colonic distension, and data acquisition in the supine and prone positions (Chen et al. 1999; Yee et al. 1999; Fenlon and Ferrucci 1997). While CTC is a relatively noninvasive imaging procedure, there are two aspects of the exam that may produce patient anxiety and potential discomfort. These include the need for bowel preparation and colonic insufflation. We stress that the colon needs to be thoroughly cleaned and properly distended to obtain an adequate examination.

As CTC technique evolves, there is a move toward standardizing techniques for performing this study. Some factors are less critical, although the best and most cost-effective alternatives are not clear. The first set of issues relate to the patient and include: the use of room air vs carbon dioxide (Dachman et al. 1998), the use of manual vs mechanical or even self-insufflation (Macari et al. 2000), the use of a routine hypotonic agent such as glucagon (Johnson and Dachman 2000), and the use of a plain catheter vs a balloon cuff catheter (Fletcher et al. 2000).

Bowel Cleansing

A more comprehensive discussion of bowel cleansing can be found in chapter 5. The minimum requirements are summarized below.

Bowel preparation is currently essential for the confident detection of lesions because residual fecal material may be indistinguishable from polyps or neoplasms, and fecal residue may obscure a polyp (Fletcher et al. 2000; Macari et al. 2001a). The radiologist should take an active role in ensuring that patients understand the importance of the preparation and what is expected of them.

There are two main bowel preparations available: cathartics such as magnesium citrate and oral phospho soda, and lavage solutions such as polyethylene glycol. In our experience, both magnesium citrate and phospho soda provide an acceptable bowel preparation. Radiologists should emphasize the need for bowel preparation and be familiar with the instructions that are provided with these commercial kits to better answer patient's questions. Magnesium citrate should not be used in patients with renal failure and phospho soda should not be used in patients with renal, cardiac, or hepatic insufficiency. We have found that the polyethylene glycol prepa-ration frequently leaves a large amount of residual fluid (Macari et al. 2001). While this preparation is adequate for colonoscopy, large amounts of residual fluid could obscure masses during CTC (whereas at conventional colonoscopy residual fluid can be aspirated out of the colon). Unlike a barium enema examination, in which different projections can be used to redistribute the fluid, in CTC the examination is usually limited to two projections, supine and prone (unless an extra view, such as a decubitus view, is obtained). In this setting, the preparation that provides the least amount of residual fluid will theoretically provide the greatest opportunity to detect polyps by enabling evaluation of the entire mucosal surface of the colon.

Getting Started

At New York University (NYU), the examination is performed entirely by a technologist or nurse. A radiologist is not on-site. Obviously, an experienced technologist or nurse is required, but after adequate training these individuals can perform the examination, minimizing the radiologist's time commitment. Conversely, at the University of Chicago all exams are performed by a radiologist. The patient is asked to evacuate the rectum immediately prior to the examination. Easy access to a nearby bathroom is essential. Some form of informed consent is used, either as required by an institutional review board or as good practice to document that this new procedure was properly explained to the patient. The exam in general takes 10 to 15 minutes of CT room time. The patient is placed on the CT table and at the radiologist's option a rectal exam may be performed. If the CT is part of a screening program offered by the radiology department without need for a referring clinician, we recommend that a digital rectal exam always be included because CTC cannot detect lesions in the anal canal.

Hypotonia

There is no objective evidence that hypotonia improves the quality of the exam (Yee et al. 1999a). After years of experience with the use of glucagon for barium enema, some radiologists believe that the added comfort is worth the expense, whereas others limit the use of glucagon to patients who experience severe cramping. When used, a 1.0-mg dose, injected intravenously over 30 seconds, is recommended. In the case of CTC, the use of glucagon has the added disadvantage of decreasing the competency of the ileocecal valve, allowing reflux of gas into the small bowel. As a result, particular attention must be paid to maximally insufflating the bowel for both the supine and prone views by adding more gas immediately prior to scanning.

Rectal Tube

Patients often have sensitive skin at the anus due to the colonic cleansing regime. Jelly, therefore, should be used to perform the rectal exam and insert the rectal tube. Too much jelly, however, may make the catheter tip too slippery. A red rubber catheter (which is smaller and may be more comfortable than a barium enema tip), a Foley catheter, or a plain barium enema tip can be used. If using a barium enema tip, barium enema tubing can be cut into 9-in strips and one end attached to the catheter tip and the other to a hand-held bulb ("blue puffer") for manual insufflation. Some investigators use a tip with a balloon cuff. The tip should be taped in place (butterfly style) to the buttock to minimize the likelihood of the tip dislodging later when the patient turns from the supine to the prone position.

Insufflation

For colonic insufflation, either room air or CO_2 can be used. We utilize air because it is easy and inexpensive. Proponents of CO_2 argue that it is readily absorbed from the colon and causes less cramping after the procedure in comparison to room air. While mild cramping may be a problem for some patients, most patients find the examination to be quick and not uncomfortable (Svensson 2002).

Air should be inflated slowly and the patient encouraged to retain the air. We ask patients to let the technologist know when they are beginning to feel discomfort from bowel distension. In general, this signals that the colon is well distended. In general, approximately 40 puffs is sufficient to distend the colon. However, we do not use a set number of puffs because the length of the human colon is variable. Also, reflex of air via an incompetent ileocecal valve will result in the need for more insufflation. It is important to be aware of the stoic patient who will wiggle their toes in silence as you puff away!

Some researchers use a mechanical pump such as a lap-aroscopic insufflator. This pump can be connected to CO_2 or compressed air. A commercial pump dedicated to CTC is also available. A set pressure setting is in general used.

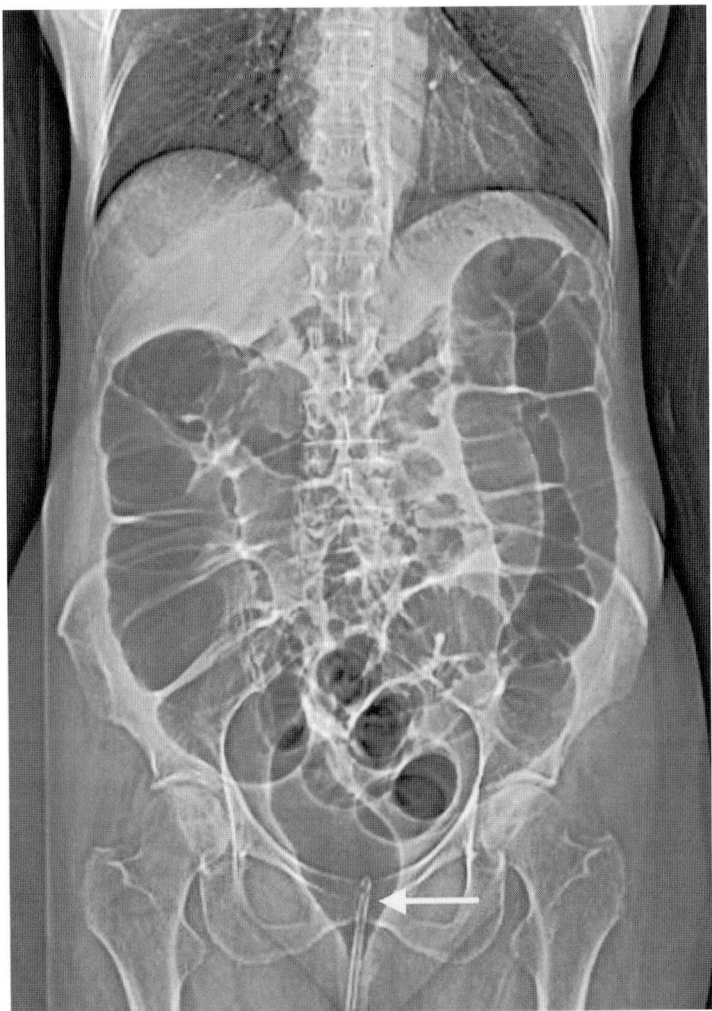

FIGURE 4.1. Adequate bowel distension. After insufflation of the colon, a scout topogram should be obtained. If the colon is distended as demonstrated here, then proceeding with data acquisition may proceed. If not, additional air insufflation is necessary. The arrow points to a thin catheter tip with no balloon permitting visualization of mucosa to the internal anal sphincter.

Performing the Scan

After insufflation, the catheter is left in the rectum and a single or biplane supine scout CT image is obtained to verify adequate bowel distension. If adequate bowel distension is present, the CT examination is performed (Fig 4.1). If adequate bowel distension is not achieved, additional air is insufflated into the rectum. Following air insufflation, CTC is performed first in the supine position in a cephalo–caudad direction encompassing the entire colon and rectum. The display field of view (DFOV) should be adjusted so as not to exclude any part of the abdomen or pelvis. That is why some technologists like to use both anteroposterior and lateral scouts. The scan range should extend several finger breaths above the top of the most cephald colon so as not to accidentally omit some colon due to a variable in the inspiration. Caudally, the scan should extend below the anal verge.

The patient is asked to hyperventilate to maximize the length of the breath hold. Some investigators use nasal oxygen, in particular in the elderly or when the technique calls for a scan longer than 30 seconds. It is best not to break up the scan into multiple breath holds. At the University of Chicago, we have found the following patient instructions to be effective in minimizing or eliminating respiratory motion: "Explain to the patient that movement of the belly will ruin the scan; take several deep breaths, as though you were going to hold your head under water. Try to hold your breath for the entire scan. If you can't, then breathe out as slowly as possibly so there will not be any rapid movement of your belly. If you must, then breathe in as slowly as possible."

As soon as the supine scan is complete, the patient is then placed in the prone position. A second scout localizing image is obtained, repeating the process over the same z-axis range. The image is reviewed to determine if the colon is adequately distended. If not, it may be necessary to insufflate scout additional gas into the colon, depending on how much the patient can tolerate. The patient is reminded that adequate distention of the bowel is critical for this study, but no additional air is insufflated into the colon against the patient's wishes.

As soon as the prone scan is complete, the catheter is positioned vertically, the puffer removed, and the rectal tip left in place. Towel or tissues should be available to cap the tubing if there is a liquid return. With the dry prep, however, there is in general little or no liquid. By finishing in the prone position and leaving the rectal tube in place open to room air for 30 to 60 seconds, postprocedure cramping should be minimized. After the tip is removed, the patient is sent to the restroom.

Supine and prone imaging doubles the radiation dose but is essential to allow optimal bowel distension, redistribution of residual fluid, and differentiation of fecal material from polyps because visualization of mobility of a filling defect implies residual fecal material. If a wet prep is used and a large amount of retained fluid is seen on the supine scan, one can optionally add a decubitus scan, optimized or tailored to move the fluid out of the loop of interest (a technique first suggested by Ken Hopper, MD, at Hershey Medical Center).

Other Technical Scan Parameters

Thin sections on a multislice scanner are strongly preferred. At NYU, we utilize a 4- × 1-mm slice detector configuration, 120 kV, 0.5-second gantry rotation, and effective 50 mAs. Pitch (table feed per gantry rotation/nominal slice thickness) should be varied between 6 and 7 such that the entire abdomen and pelvis may be covered during a 30-second breath hold. The pitch is varied to account for differences in patient's body length so that the acquisition can be completed in 30 seconds. This results in 12 and 14 mm of coverage per second. CT images are reconstructed as 1.25-mm-thick sections with a 1-mm reconstruction interval. The examination is networked to a workstation for interpretation.

At the University of Chicago, we use a 1.25-mm collimation, 7.5-mm/sec table speed, HS (high-speed) mode, with overlapping reconstructions to 1.0 mm, kV = 120, mA = 100, and soft algorithm (GE LightSpeed, GE Medical Systems). Nasal oxygen is used for scans longer than 30 seconds.

Regardless of the scanner type, it must be stressed that interpretation of multiplanar reformations (MPR) and 3D endoluminal data is facilitated by thin section (<3 mm) image acquisition (Fig 4.2.). If one does not own a multislice scanner, in our opinion, the thickest acceptable sections are 2.5 mm with a pitch = 1.5, and overlapping reconstruction to 1 to 1.5 mm.

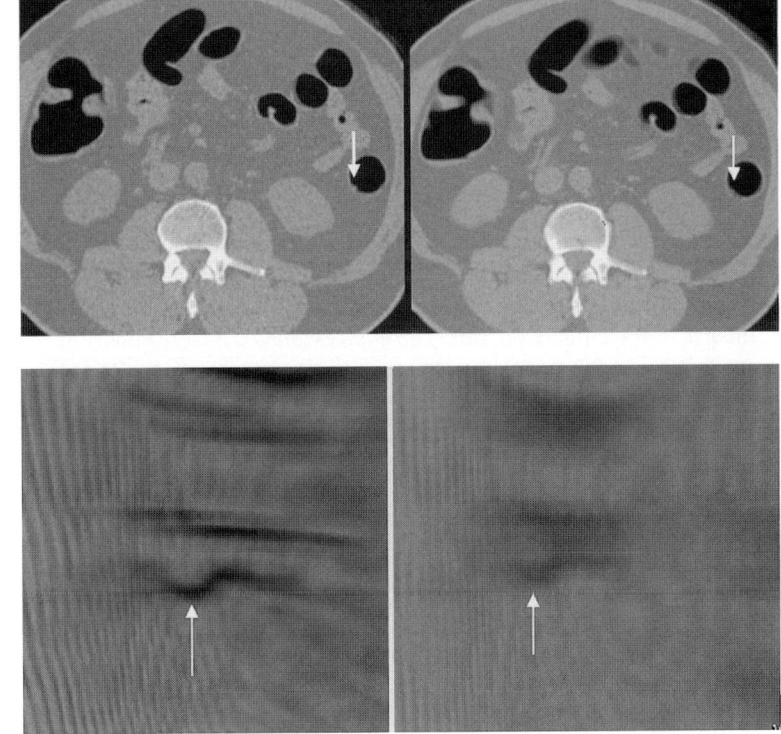

FIGURE 4.2. Effect of slice thickness (1.25 mm vs 5.0 mm) on image quality. (A) Axial CT images reconstructed from same data set using 4- × 1-mm detector configuration. The image on the left is reconstructed as a 1.25-mm-thick slice with 1-mm overlap. The image on the right is reconstructed as a 5-mm-thick slice with 2.5-mm overlap. In both images, arrows point to a 3-mm polyp in the descending colon, which is seen with less volume averaging with the thin slice (left). (B) Same data set now with 3D endoluminal perspective. Because of less volume averaging, the polyp (arrow) is clearly seen with the 1.25-mm data set (arrow) but almost imperceptible with the thicker slice (right).

Management and Interpretation of CT Data

Once the CT examination is completed, the data is transferred to a workstation that allows fast, seamless interaction of axial, MPR, and 3D endoluminal images. This is essential for data interpretation. At the same time, it should be recognized that networking data to an appropriate workstation may be time consuming given the large number of images that are generated with thin-section studies.

Once the CT data are on the workstation, the primary question is whether to begin interpretation using a 2D or 3D technique. This choice is influenced by personal preference and the available workstation and features of the software package used. While there are advocates for both techniques, and hardware and software will surely improve, most researchers currently utilize a primary 2D approach with MPR and 3D imaging reserved for problem solving (Dachman et al. 1998; Macari et al. 2001a; Johnson and Dachman 2000; Fletcher et al. 2000). Novel display methods are still under investigation (see chapter 6).

Why 2D Imaging?

The main rationale for interpreting CTC using a primary 2D approach is speed of interpretation. At the time of this writing (February 2001) our interpretation time is 5 to 20 minutes, often less than 10 minutes. For CTC to be a clinically viable tool in everyday radiology practice, the examination needs to be performed and interpreted in a "time-efficient" manner. While technologists can be trained to perform colonic insufflation (saving radiologist time), they cannot interpret axial images. For example, in 2001 Yee et al. evaluated a large cohort of patients using both 2D and 3D imaging (with antegrade and retrograde 3D colon navigation) in both the supine and prone positions. In this study, the median interpretation times for two different radiologists were 31 minutes (range of 15 to 45 minutes) and 27 minutes (range of 15 to 40 minutes), respectively (Yee et al. 2001). The sensitivity for CT for polyps 10 mm and larger was over 90%. However, results reported in this study were based on a consensus interpretation and, after factoring in the time for consensus, a significant amount of radiologist time was probably spent in evaluating these colonography data sets by consensus. This time issue is especially relevant with the introduction of multislice CTC in which close to 1000 images can be obtained per patient, depending on slice collimation and degree of overlap.

Dachman et al. (1998) reported findings in 44 patients using 2D imaging with 3D imaging for problem solving. In this study of two radiologists, the sensitivity for polyps larger than 8 mm was 83% and the specificity was 100% for both observers. The average amount of time spent on interpretation was 28 minutes, 30 seconds (range of 14 to 65 minutes). Macari et al. (2001c) reported findings for a similar approach using primary axial 2D imaging with 3D and MPR for problem solving only. In that study, 42 patients undergoing colonoscopy screening were examined with CT immediately before endoscopy. Data were interpreted by two different radiologists using one of two methods. In method 1, axial 2D data sets were examined in a cine mode at a workstation. Only if findings were suggestive of an abnormality were those areas examined with MPR and 3D CT techniques in an attempt to differentiate residual fecal material and folds from polyps. In method 2, data sets were examined exactly as in method 1 and, subsequent to that review, data were examined with 3D "fly-through" endoluminal navigation and multiplanar reformatted images. Using method 1, the mean evaluation time was 16 minutes. With method 2, the mean evaluation time was 40 minutes. No additional polyps were detected with method 2.

As experience with 2D imaging as a primary interpretation technique has increased, the time required to evaluate colonography data sets has decreased. The reason for this is that as reader experience in differentiating bulbous folds and residual fecal material from polyps increases, the frequency of MPR and 3D utilization for problem solving decreases. Also, workstations have faster processors and greater memory. A recent study evaluating multislice CTC in colorectal polyp detection using a primary 2D technique showed the mean time of CT data interpretation was 11 minutes (range of 7 to 20 minutes), with a median time of 12 minutes for complete supine and prone evaluation (Macari et al. 2001c). In this study, CT sensitivity for polyps larger 10 mm was 93%.

In general, examinations can be interpreted more quickly in well-prepared patients with little residual fluid or fecal material in whom no polyps are present because MPR and 3D imaging for problem solving are required less frequently. Colons that are redundant or contain polyps and residual fecal material require longer interpretation times.

Evaluation of the entire colon in 2D is facilitated by a workstation that allows a rapid scrolling or cine through the colon. Because the colon is not a straight tube but rather a tortuous redundant organ, it is imperative that up-and-down scrolling be performed so that the entire colon is evaluated. The easiest approach is to start in the rectum and proceed in a retrograde direction to the cecum.

The layout of images on the screen is a user option. Some of our favorite choices are:

1. Use a full-screen view of the axial image, paging with either a mouse (go slowly!) or a key to page one image at a time (Dachman et al. 1998). Toggle to MPRs or 3D as needed.
2. A four-on-one view showing both supine and prone axial images simultaneously (they can be synchronized and linked) with one MPR (usually a coronal view) at the same time (Macari et al. 2001). One can toggle to the 3D view as needed. Many software programs permit problem solving of multiple "bookmarked" areas all at once, at the end of your review.
3. If your software will not show simultaneous prone and supine images, use 4-on-1 axial, coronal, sagittal, and oblique MPRs of one patient position at a time (Johnson et al. 2000).

Another advantage of this approach is that you are guaranteed to see 100% of the scanned mucosal surface, unlike a primary endoluminal read in which some mucosa is obscured.

In summary, it appears that reliance upon a primary 2D interpretation technique, with MPR and 3D imaging used for problem solving only, allows data to be interpreted in a time-efficient manner with excellent sensitivity (>90%) for polyps ≥10 mm (Dachman et al. 1998; Macari et al. 2001c, Johnson and Dachman 2000) (Figs 4.3 and 4.4).

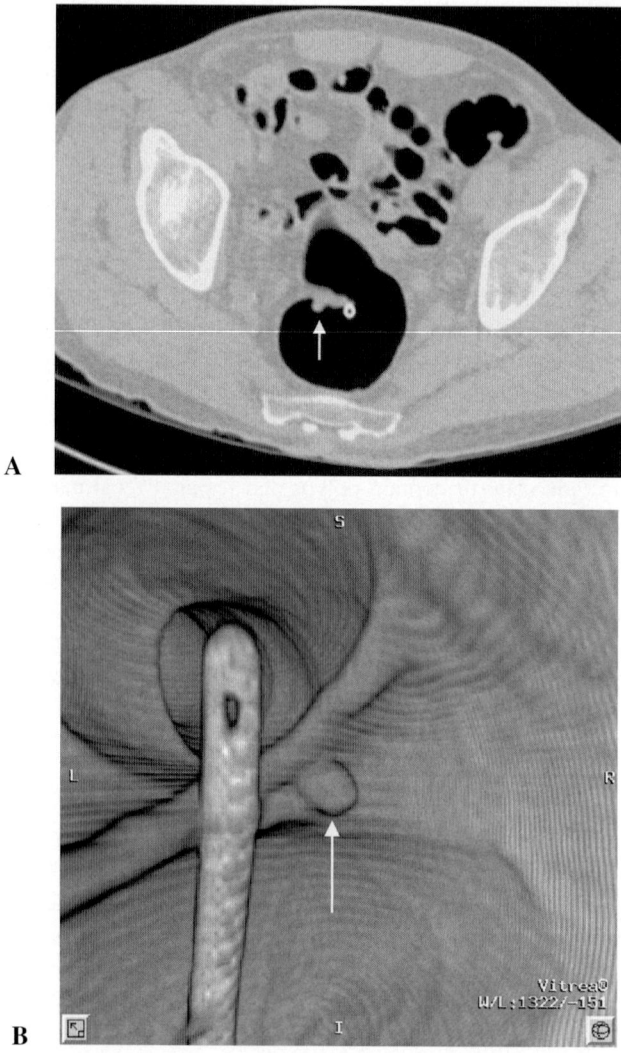

FIGURE 4.3. Seventy-five-year-old man with an adenoma arising on a rectal fold. (**A**) Axial CT scan of rectum shows 8-mm filling defect (arrow) suspicious for polyp. Note that the filling defect is homogeneous in attenuation without bubbles of gas or internal heterogeneity. (**B**) Three-dimensional volume-rendered endoluminal image of the rectum confirms the polypoid morphology of the filling defect (arrow). At colonoscopy, an 8-mm tubular adenoma was removed.

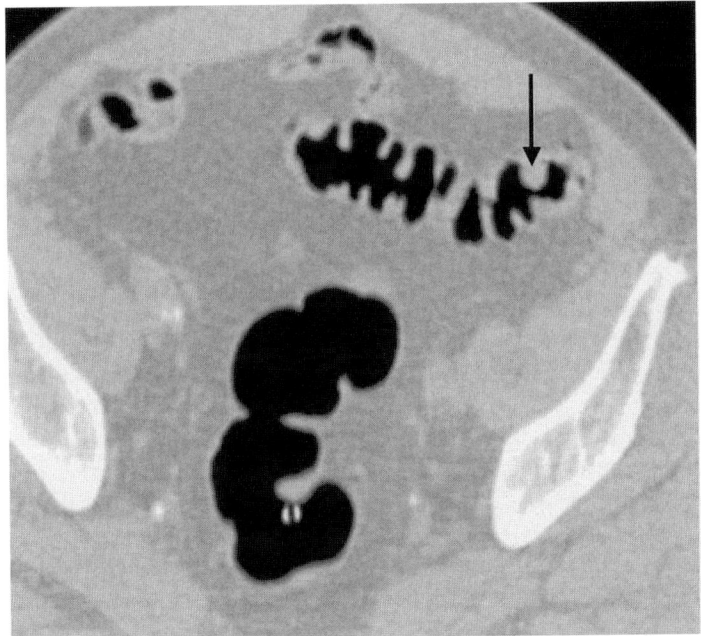

A

B

FIGURE 4.4. Value of multiplanar reconstructions. (**A**) Axial CT scan of sigmoid shows a 9-mm lobular filling defect (arrow) suspicious for polyp in a moderately distended sigmoid colon with some muscular hypertrophy. (**B**) Coronal image shows that this has linear morphology (arrow) consistent with an interhaustral fold.

Why 3D Imaging?

Primary reliance on 3D "virtual colonoscopy" techniques has the appeal of truly simulating conventional colonoscopy. Several workstation vendors using either surface- or volume-rendered images are incorporating a centerline that the computer will generate automatically followed by a movie of the endoluminal view traversing this centerline. One can then navigate through the colon, either forward or backward, and stop to evaluate suspicious abnormalities. Optimization of review parameters such as threshold and lighting are software specifics and for the purpose of this discussion we will assume they have been optimized.

Limitations are encountered when segments of the colon are not well distended and the centerline cannot be generated. On occasion, in overdistended segments the centerline may jump to an adjacent distended loop of large or small bowel. Moreover, most workstations that incorporate a 3D viewing technique do not ensure that the entire colonic surface is evaluated. Another limitation of primary 3D imaging (like primary 2D imaging) is that it cannot be used as the sole technique for data evaluation. Using a 3D technique may result in many false positives. Just as 3D imaging and MPR imaging are used for problem solving when 2D imaging is the primary interpretation technique, so is 2D imaging used as a problem solver for 3D imaging (Macari et al. 2001). This is to aid in evaluation of attenuation characteristics of lesions as well as evaluation of filling defects that are mural or extrinsic in origin. Often lesions detected with 3D CTC techniques may have morphological features suggestive of a polyp or neoplasm. When these same areas are evaluated with 2D CT, however, a variety of normal structures (including fecal material and extrinsic defects) may be found to have simulated the abnormalities visualized with 3D rendering (Macari et al. 2001). Finally, as stated above, the amount of time for data evaluation using these 3D techniques may limit its use in a clinical setting. Primary 3D imaging techniques need to become faster and more automated with ease of navigation before they can be relied upon as a primary viewing technique.

Despite these limitations, it is possible that by evaluating 3D endoluminal images, both antegrade and retrograde, smaller polyps (<5 mm) can be routinely detected. A recent study found that using axial images, as well as complete 3D endoluminal navigation in antegrade and retrograde directions in both the supine and prone positions, detection of polyps ≤ 5 mm was 59% (Yee et al. 2001). This compares favorably to a recent report in which 2D imaging was used as the primary data interpretation technique (Macari et al. 2002). In this study, using a primary 2D technique, less than 20% of the diminutive polyps were visualized. However, the detection of these diminutive polyps is of questionable clinical significance, especially if routine colon screening is to be performed on an interval basis (Macari et al. 2000; Glick et al. 1998). A recent study showed that the majority (68%) of polyps ≤ 5 mm that were missed using a primary 2D technique were either hyperplastic polyps or normal colon at pathology (Macari et al. 2002). Thirty percent were small tubular adenomas. This underscores the point that colon screening is not a one-time event. However, it should also be stressed that colon screening examination is 100% sensitive for these small polyps and they may be missed even at colonoscopy (Rex et al. 1997).

How Should the Data Be Interpreted?

Optimal evaluation of CTC data sets are facilitated by easy access to supine and prone images and 2D and 3D images. Several workstations allow both the axial supine and prone images to be displayed adjacent to each other. In a screening population where the prevalence of polyps is low, this may be the optimal approach for data interpretation. Having easy access to both data sets assures that segments of the colon that are filled with fluid or incompletely distended on one data set are free of fluid and well distended on the other (Chen et al. 1999; Macari et al. 2001c) (Fig 4.5). In general, however, even in a screening population it

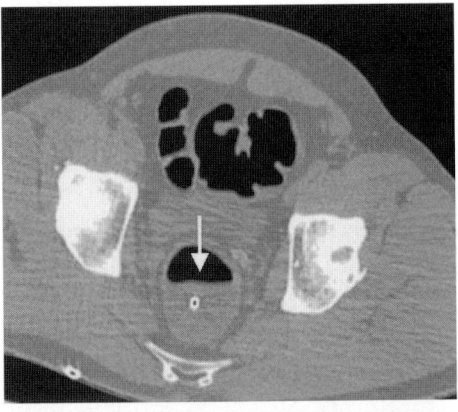

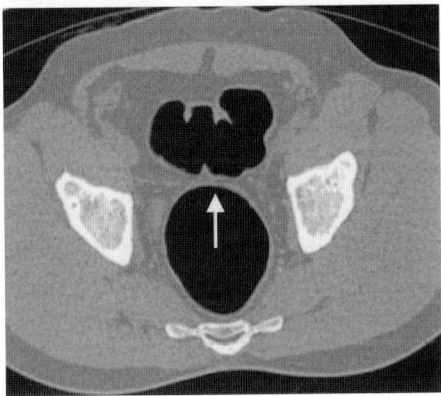

FIGURE 4.5. Effect of positioning and redistribution of fluid. The image on the top shows supine image of the rectum with a large amount of residual fluid (arrow). The image on the bottom is the prone view of the same location showing *all walls of the* rectum without fluid because of redistribution.

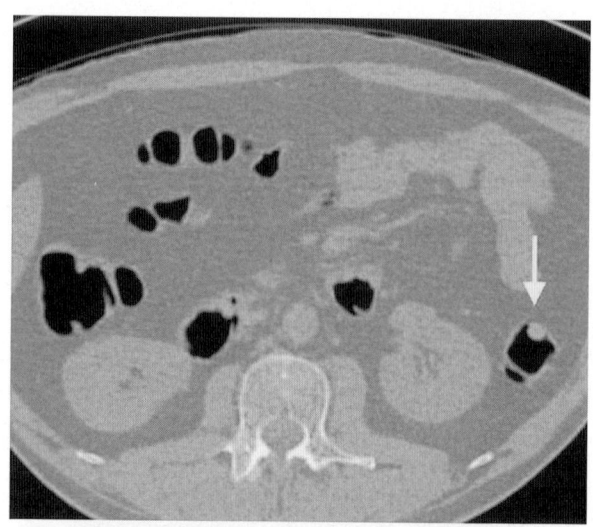

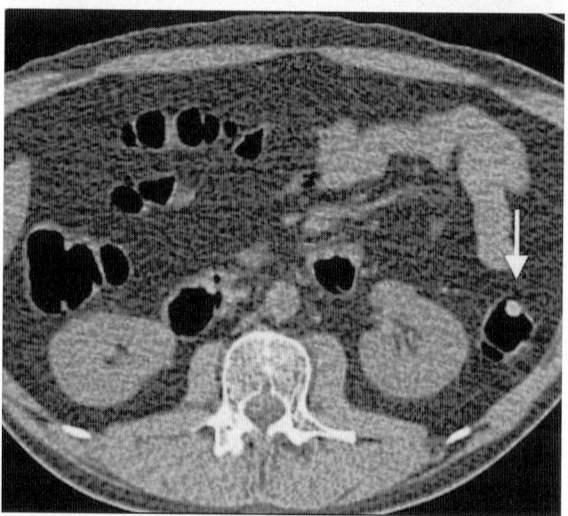

FIGURE 4.6. Effect of changing window-level settings. The image on the top shows a prone CT image of the descending colon using wide W/L settings with filling defect suspicious for polyp (arrow). The image on the bottom shows the same location with narrow W/L settings. It can be seen that this has central high attenuation and therefore is not a polyp (arrow).

will be necessary in a substantial percentage of cases to evaluate suspected abnormalities visualized on 2D imaging. Therefore, in addition to the supine and prone axial data sets, quick interaction of suspected abnormalities with MPR and 3D imaging to evaluate these areas is necessary. Moreover, being able to rapidly change window/level settings from wide to narrow facilitates data interpretation (Fig 4.6).

Below is an overview of the appearance of the normal colon and how to differentiate residual fecal material, bulbous folds, and polyps using a combination of 2D and 3D techniques. These issues are dealt with in part 2 of this atlas as well.

Normal Colon

Adequate insufflation with gas (either room air or CO_2 gas) results in a well-distended colon. Depending on the degree of distension, the appearance of the normal colonic lumen will vary with 3D rendering. The mucosa will appear relatively featureless if the interhaustral folds are completely effaced by the pressure of the gas (Fig 4.7). This featureless appearance is more often detected in the descending colon and rectum where the haustra are relatively sparse (Blackstone 1984). In the cecum, as well as the ascending, transverse, and sigmoid colon, thin curvilinear interhaustral folds will be visualized either randomly oriented or evenly spaced along the colonic surface. The colon wall typically has a circular contour when well distended (Fig 4.7). In the transverse colon, the appearance on the endoluminal view may be more triangular in configuration (Blackstone 1984) (Fig 4.8).

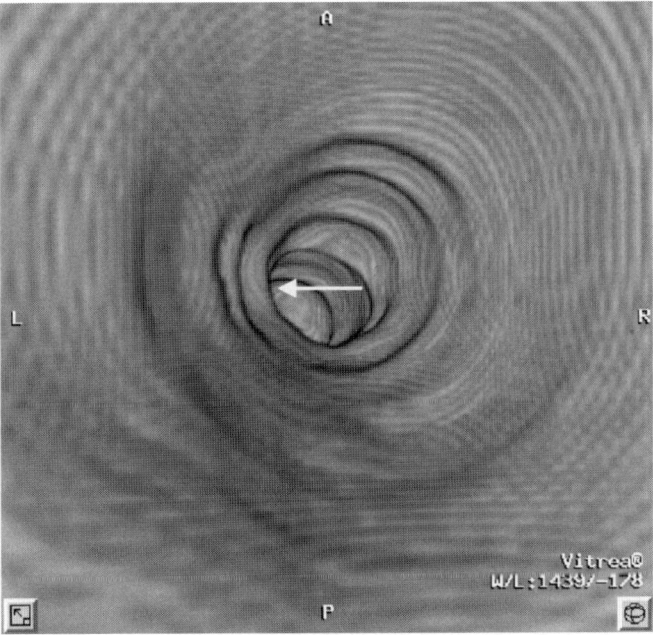

FIGURE 4.7. Normal endoluminal view of sigmoid/descending colon junction. In the foreground the folds are effaced by the pressure of the distension, giving a relatively featureless appearance. In the more distal aspect of this view, several delicate folds are visualized (arrow).

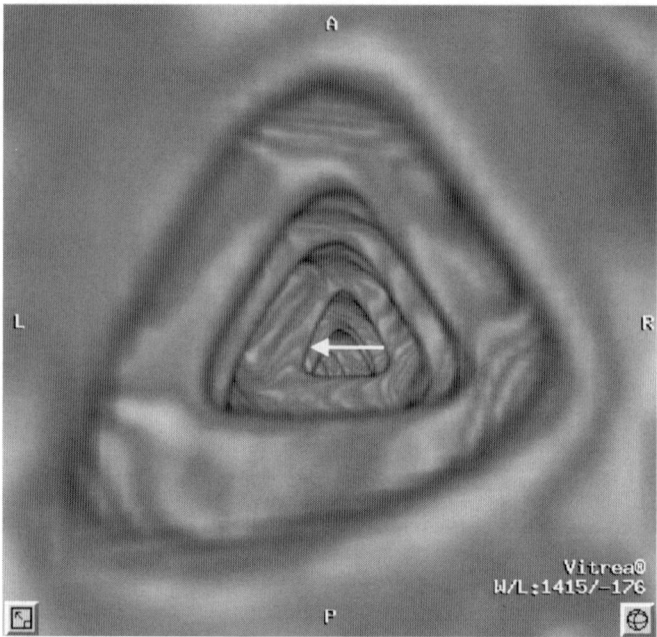

FIGURE 4.8. Normal endoluminal view of the transverse colon. The transverse colon usually has a triangular appearance. Note interhaustral folds (arrow).

Regardless of the method of the primary reading, a 3D barium-enema-like view is ideal for display of the polyp location and measurement of distance from the anal canal. Also, the measurement of polyp size is best done using the 2D data. This is important because size threshold may determine whether the radiologist recommends follow-up vs colonoscopy.

If the colon is not properly distended, 3D endoluminal visualization will be limited and adequate rendering may not be possible (Fig 4.9). Inadequate distention most often occurs in the sigmoid, especially when there is muscular hypertrophy and severe diverticular disease. In some cases, it may be impossible to evaluate this region. Flexible sigmoidoscopy or colonoscopy should be recommended, depending on the portion of bowel not adequately evaluated by CT.

When evaluating the colon with a 3D endoluminal technique, a circumferential constricting neoplasm may be difficult to distinguish from a collapsed segment (Fig 4.10). Visualization of an irregular, nonsmooth surface may be the only clue to the presence of such a lesion.

It is often easier to recognize the lesion with 2D imaging, either axial or MPR images. When a neoplasm is identified, a search for adenopathy (on soft-tissue windows) and liver metastases (on narrow windows) should be performed. In addition, polyps are more difficult to perceive in collapsed segments.

In general, adequate distension is recognized by obtaining a scout image after colonic insufflation. If distension appears adequate, the patient is scanned. After

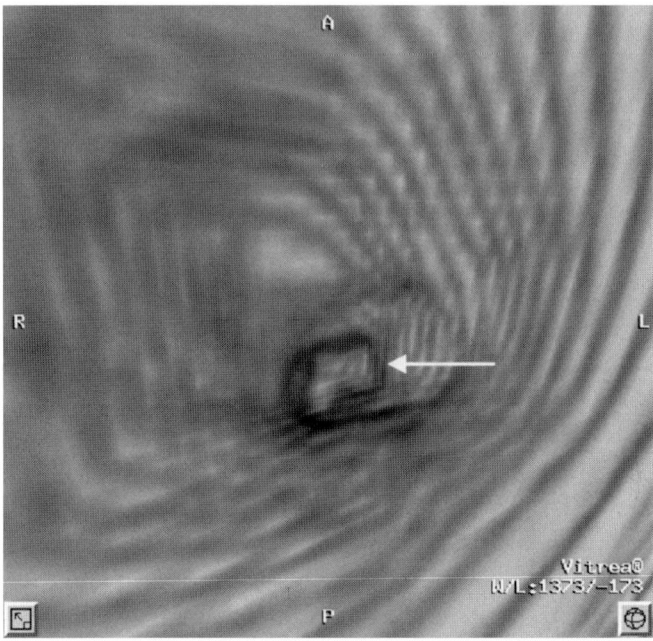

FIGURE 4.9. Endoluminal view of collapsed colon. When the colon is collapsed, endoluminal navigation is impossible. This view shows colon is occluded from collapse (arrow). Please compare to Fig 4.10.

the data set is obtained, the degree of distension is better appreciated on 2D images than on 3D images. Several workstations allow a simulation of a double-contrast barium enema image, which allows a quick overview of how well the colon is distended to facilitate polyp location (probably with greater accuracy than colonoscopy).

Residual Fecal Material

The major interpretative pitfall with either 2D or 3D evaluation is mistaking residual fecal material for a polyp or neoplasm. The colon needs to be rigorously cleansed prior to CTC. However, even in compliant patients, small amounts of residual fecal material may persist. There are a number of techniques that facilitate differentiation of residual fecal material from true polyps. Most fecal debris will remain on the dependent surface of the bowel when the patient is moved from the supine to the prone position (Fig 4.11). On occasional, howeer, fecal material will be adherent to the wall and will not change position. In these cases, differentiation of polyp from fecal material is facilitated by the acquisition of thin-section CTC.

To obtain thin-section CTC, a multidetector-row CT scanner is necessary. The main advantage of performing CTC with thin sections (either 4- × 1- or 1.25-mm slices) is that near isotropic voxels are available for data review. De-

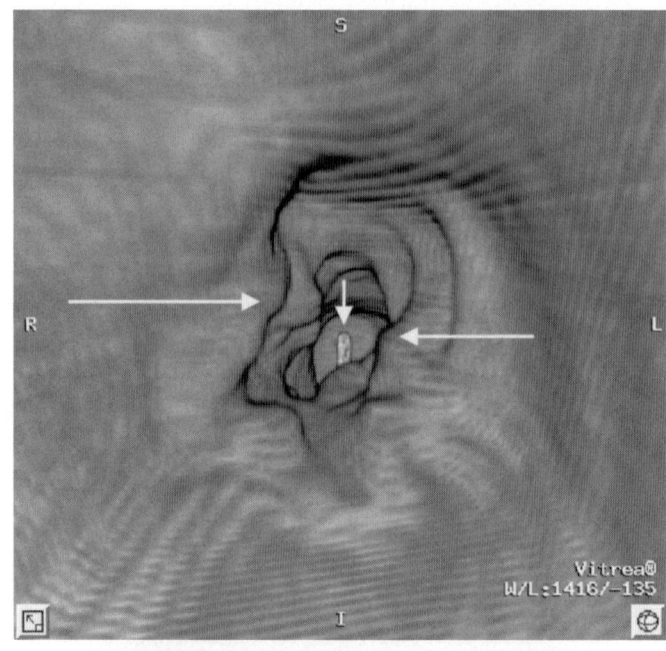

A

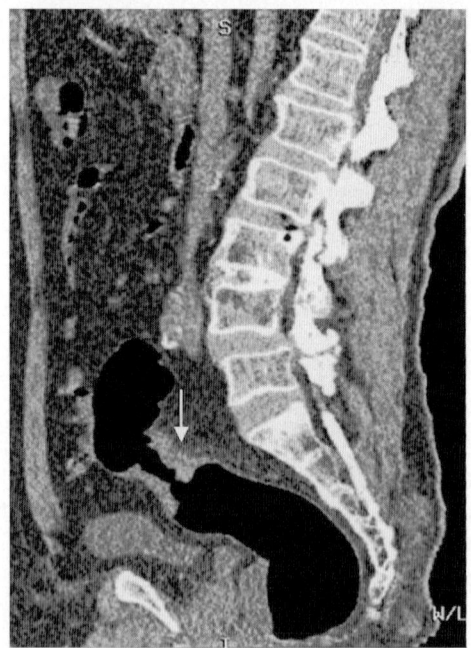

B

FIGURE 4.10. Sixty-five-year-old man undergoing virtual colonoscopy with partially constricting adenocarcinoma. (**A**) 3D endoluminal view of sigmoid colon shows irregular folds in the colon (long arrows). Note rectal catheter in background (short arrow). (**B**) Sagittal image shows better the "apple-core" appearance of the neoplasm (arrow).

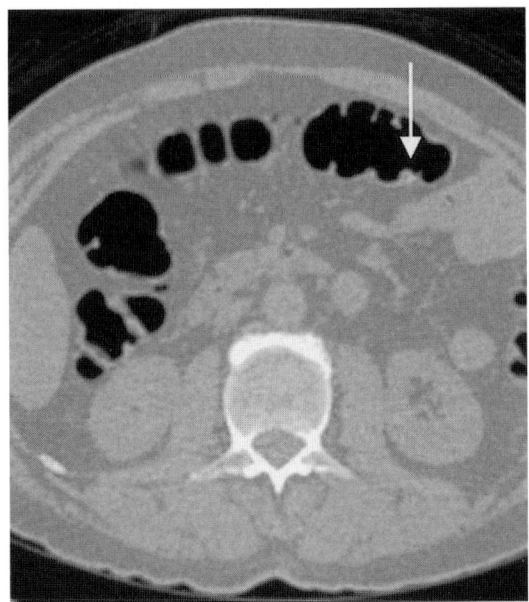

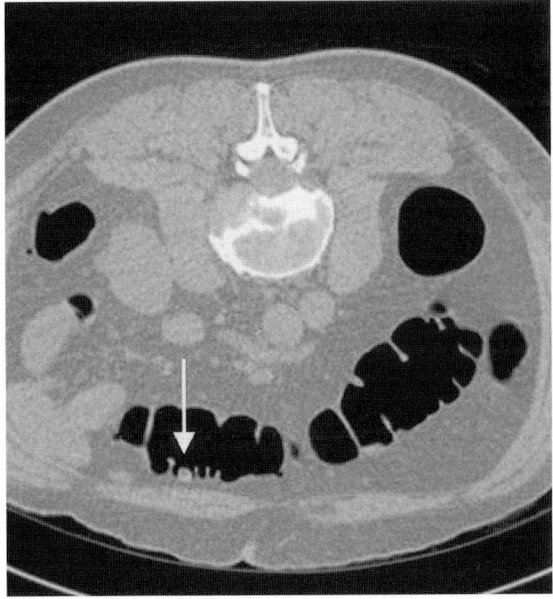

FIGURE 4.11. Mobile filling defect consistent with stool (arrow). The axial CT image on the left shows a small round filling defect in the transverse colon on the dorsal surface (arrow). When the patient is turned prone (right), the filling defect is now noted to be on the ventral surface (arrow).

pending on the field of view used, the z-axis pixel dimension (1 mm) is only slightly greater than the x- and y-axis pixel dimensions. We have found that the major advantage of thin-section multidetector-row CT has been a decreased number of false positive studies. The majority of false positive findings at CTC are due to poor patient preparation, poor colonic distention, and bulbous haustral folds (Fletcher et al. 2000; Yee et al. 2001; Hara et al. 2001). A high false positive rate may decrease the utility of virtual colonoscopy, as many unnecessary colonoscopies will be required. When compared to thicker slices, the potential advantages of obtaining near isotropic voxels for CTC include improved morphological analysis of suspected lesions seen on axial images, much better z-axis resolution for multiplanar reformats and 3D viewing, and better evaluation of internal attenuation (gas bubbles, areas of high density, or homogenous soft-tissue attenuation) within detected filling defects (Fig 4.12). Because there is less volume averaging within a thin-collimation CT slice when compared to thicker sections, detection and visualization of small bubbles of gas or high-attenuation material within detected filling defects is facilitated. The finding of internal heterogeneities (either high or low attenuating) within the central portion of small colonic filling defects is consistent with residual fecal material rather than polyps (Fig 4.6).

It must be stressed that both 3D (surface and volume) rendering techniques currently in use for endoluminal display are not sensitive to the presence of this air or high-attenuation material; however, air and high-attenuation material are readily apparent on the 2D images (especially with narrow window-level settings), underscoring the need to correlate 2D and 3D information. Residual barium within the fecal material may help differentiate stool from neoplasms. There is currently interest in developing orally ingested bowel preparations that would "label" residual fecal material with barium, potentially aiding in the differentiation of stool from polyps (Fenlon et al. 1999).

In addition to mobility and internal attenuation characteristics, morphological analysis can be helpful in differentiating residual fecal material from polyps. Polyps and small tumors have round or lobulated smooth borders, whereas residual fecal material often contains irregular geometric angled borders and edges. By utilizing thin-section CT, the smooth or geometric morphology of a filling defect can be better investigated on both 2D and 3D endoluminal views. Recognizing these features of adherent fecal material should decrease the false positive rate.

Bulbous Folds

A second major pitfall of CTC interpretation is differentiating bulbous irregular folds from polyps. Improved z-axis resolution with thin-section multidetector-row CT facilitates differentiation of bulbous folds from polyps. On axial review, a bulbous fold may appear as a pedunculated polyp (Fig 4.4). However, careful inspection of MPR and endoluminal images usually allows differentiation of linear (fold) morphology from true polypoid morphology. While polypoid morphology on 3D imaging may represent stool or a polyp (Figs 4.3 and 4.5), lin-

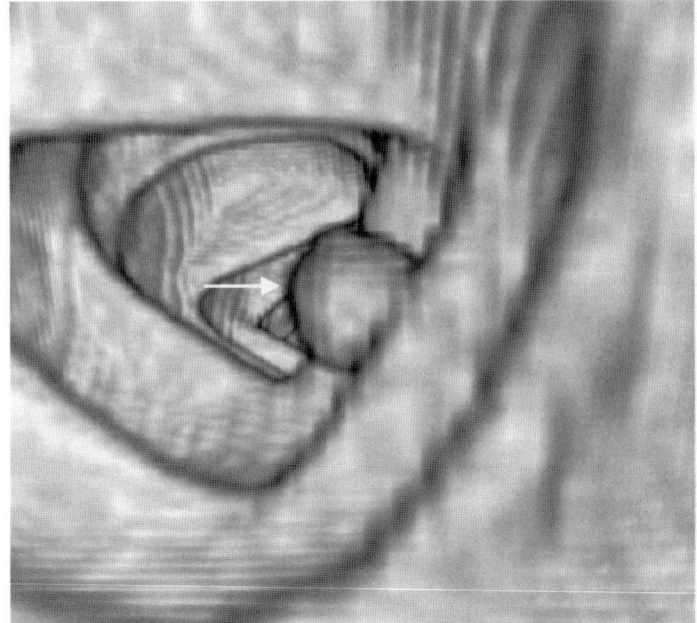

A

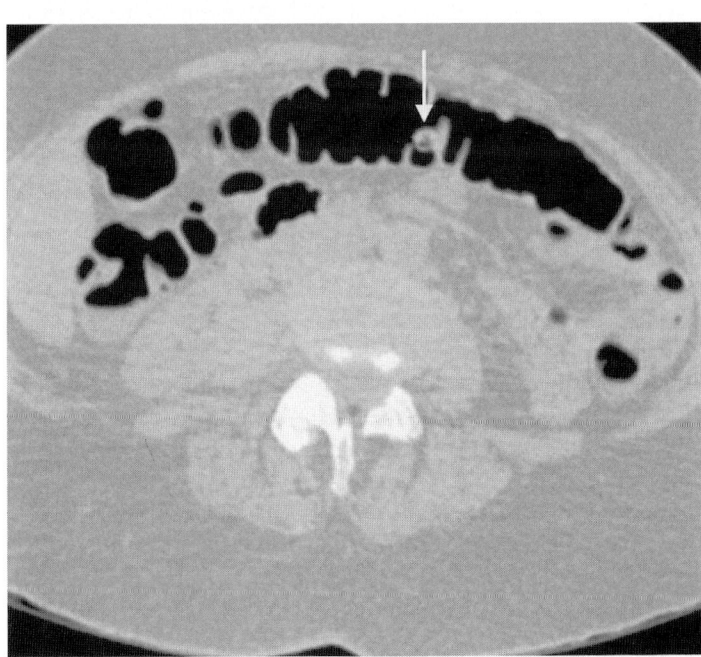

B

FIGURE 4.12. Primary 3D read with 2D problem solving in a dependent, 58-year-old man undergoing virtual colonoscopy. (A) 3D endoluminal view shows a polypoid-filling defect in the transverse colon (arrow). Differential diagnosis includes polyp and residual stool. (B) Axial CT image shows small bubbles of gas centrally within filling defect, confirming residual fecal material (arrow).

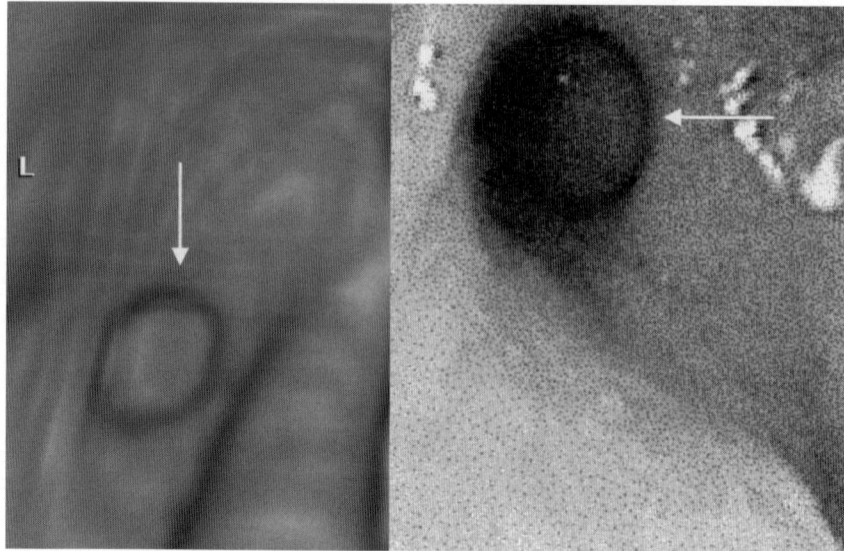

FIGURE 4.13. Diverticulum on endoluminal view (left) shows a *complete* ring around the diverticulum (arrow). The image on the right confirms the colonoscopic view of the same diverticulum (arrow). Compare its appearance with the polyp in Fig 4.3, where there is *not* a complete ring.

ear morphology is indicative of a fold. On occasion, bulbous folds can be difficult to differentiate from polyps. If there is concern, and the lesion is of substantial size (as measured on the 2D image), colonoscopy is recommended for differentiation in these cases.

Diverticula

Diverticula may simulate polyps on 3D endoluminal displays (Fig 4.13A). A diverticulum will be noted to have a dense ring around it identifying the orifice (Macari et al.; Fenlon et al. 1998). In contrast, a polyp does not have a complete ring shadow surrounding it, as it is a raised structure (Fig 4.13B). When a diverticulum is impacted with fecal material, it may appear raised, mimicking a polyp. In these cases, 2D imaging is necessary to show both the higher density within the impacted diverticulum as well as the portion of the diverticulum extending outside the colonic wall.

Ileocecal Valve

Three appearances of the normal ileocecal valve have been characterized by colonoscopists: a papillary type, with a dome-like protrusion with its mouth at the apex; a labial type, appearing as a slightly raised fold with the mouth separating the fold margins; and an intermediate type (Blackstone 1984). Differentiating the valve from neoplasm is usually not difficult because the valve has a characteristic location. However, the morphological appearance of the ileocecal valve at 3D CTC may be similar to that of a polyp or neoplasm. Two-dimensional axial or MPR evaluation allows the terminal ileum to be evaluated, which can then be followed directly to the valve (Fig 4.14). Often, the ileocecal valve contains adipose tissue, facilitating its identification.

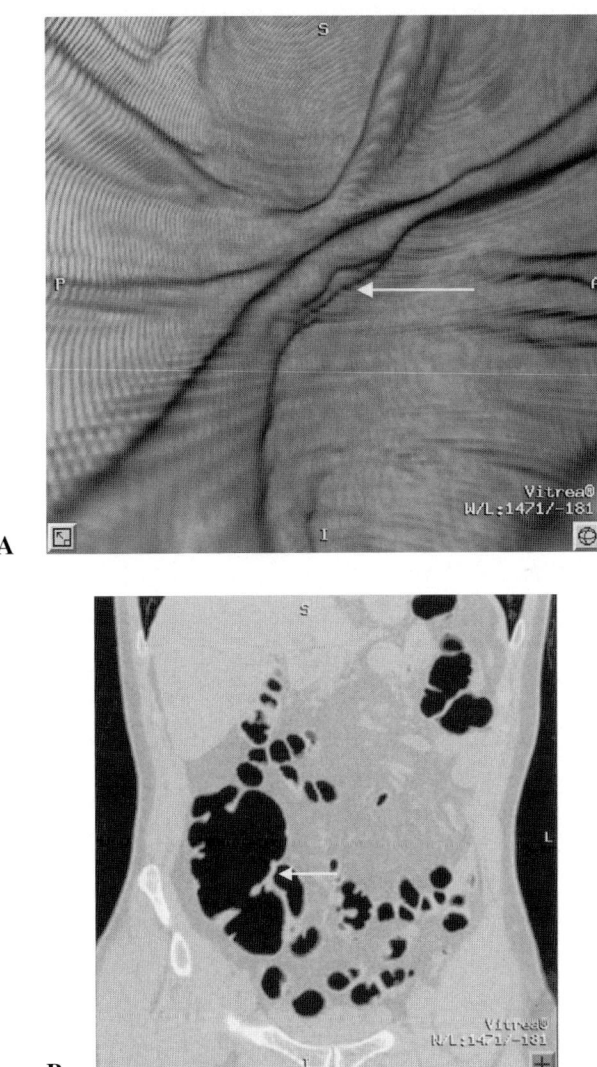

FIGURE 4.14. Ileocecal valve. (**A**) 3D endoluminal view shows polypoid-filling defect in the cecum (arrow). Morphology is most consistent with the ileocecal valve. However, masses can occur on or near the valve, so 2D confirmation is helpful. (**B**) Coronal CT image shows terminal ileum entering the cecum at this level, confirming ileocecal valve (arrow).

Extrinsic Defects

Any organ or structure that is outside the colon can cause external compression of the bowel. Because extrinsic structures usually compress the colon along a focal area of the distended colon, they do not appear as occlusive lesions. Rather, when evaluated from an endoluminal 3D perspective, these external structures compressing the wall may appear to represent focal neoplasms. We have noted external compression from the liver, other loops of bowel, the psoas muscle, and aorta. Similar external compression effects may be detected related to the spleen and kidneys. These external compressions may be more common in thin patients, underscoring the need for 2D correlation whenever an abnormality is detected on 3D.

Future Developments

See Chapter 6 for novel display techniques and chapter 8 for computer-aided diagnosis.

5

Patient Preparation

Michael Zalis

As is the case with many radiological examinations, computer tomography (CT) colonography (CTC) requires adequate preparation of the patient prior to imaging to achieve its full diagnostic potential. Properly performed, the preparatory steps of CTC contribute to high sensitivity for detection of polyps and can be obtained with a minimum of patient discomfort. In this chapter, we will focus on two topics central to achieving a high-quality exam: patient education and bowel preparation. Our review will include methods currently employed to achieve these ends, as well as a discussion of research aimed at improving them. Throughout this chapter, we will emphasize practical aspects of patient preparation that can improve both patient comfort and the quality of colonography images.

Patient Education

Patients often experience considerable anxiety as they approach colon examinations, in part due to their expectation of perceived embarrassment and discomfort (Weitzman 2001). This expectation of discomfort contributes to the relatively low compliance rate of individuals for recommended colon cancer screening regimens (Brown et al. 1990). Therefore, steps that reduce patient anxiety and improve patient comfort will likely contribute to the larger goal of improving compliance for colon cancer screening. For the individual patient, the clinician can provide information to appropriately set the patient's expectations about the procedure, thereby contributing to the ease of performance and quality of the exam.

As a first step to reducing anxiety, the clinician can assure the prospective patient that CTC is easily tolerated. For the vast majority of patients, CTC is associated with no or at most mild discomfort (Fenlon et al. 1999). Eighty-two percent of patients surveyed in a clinical trial comparing CTC to colonoscopy who reported a binary preference for one exam chose CTC over endoscopy, despite the fact that colonoscopy is performed with intravenous (IV) anesthetic and amnesic medications while CTC is not (Svensson et al. 2001). Seventy percent of patients in the same trial reported the discomfort associated with CTC as "not unpleasant" or "slightly unpleasant" (Svensson et al. 2002). In addition, because no conscious sedation or monitoring is required, there is no need for an IV line to perform CTC. While compared to other interventions the placement of an IV line may seem trivial, it is important to remember that the majority of individuals for whom screening is recommended are otherwise healthy, and every inconvenience may be construed as a potential contributing factor for poor compliance.

While easily tolerated, CTC is not completely pain free for all individuals. Approximately 5% of patients report some degree of bowel cramping with insufflation of the colon. In our experience, this is associated with moderate discomfort at most. In all instances, the cramping resolves spontaneously within 1 to 2 hours. Unfortunately, little data are available for either first-encounter or returning patients to predict which will experience cramping discomfort. In a 4-year experience with over 200 exams, we have yet to observe severe or debilitating discomfort associated with CTC as reported by our patients.

As both the CT and magnetic resonance imaging (MRI) versions of colonography involve high-resolution imaging of the abdomen, some form of breathing suspension is required for each (Fenlon et al. 1999; Luboldt et al. 1998; Debatin et al. 1999; Fletcher and Luboldt 2000). In the case of CTC, the length of breath suspension depends on the size of the patient and the type of scanner employed. For a typical adult, the superior-to-inferior coverage required to image the colon is approximately 36 cm. If performed on a multidetector helical scanner, this translates into an acquisition time of approximately 20 seconds per prone or supine series. For the majority of patients, 20 seconds is an acceptable length of time to hold one's breath. For single-detector helical scanners, this scan length is usually unacceptably long for a single-breath hold (greater than 30 seconds). When performing CTC on single-detector scanners, several investigators have achieved high-quality examinations by instructing patients to suspend breathing only for the first portion of each exam series and to resume spontaneous breathing as they see fit (Dachman et al. 1998; Fenlon et al. 1999). If the scan protocol begins near the liver dome and continues inferiorly, the result of the temporary breath suspension instruction is that breathing artifact is reduced for portions of the colon near the diaphragm. As scanning continues into the pelvis and the patient resumes breathing, images of the inferior portions of the colon are relatively unaffected by shallow diaphragmatic excursion.

Scan protocols for MRI colonography are typically designed around either extremely fast, non-breath–hold sequences, such as the single-shot turbo spin echo protocol, or a series of gradient T_1- and turbo spin echo T_2-weighted sequences (Luboldt et al. 1998; Debatin et al. 1999; Morrin et al. 2001). In each case, imaging sequences are designed with scan times less than 25 seconds per series, an acceptable duration for most patients. Hence, for current protocols of colonography involving both CT and MRI, patients can be reassured that they will not have to endure prolonged or anxiety-provoking suspension of breathing.

Patients can also be informed that the typical CTC is a brief procedure. In our experience, once the patient is changed and escorted to the scanner room the exam can be completed within 15 minutes. Most of this time is used in the placement of the rectal tube and insufflation of air into the colon. As described briefly above, the image acquisition sequences are relatively short, and there is no required recovery period, per se, following the exam. The result is that most patients can expect to be fully functional immediately after the procedure. Patients should be able to drive and may return to home or work without observation or convalescence.

Bowel Preparation

The current technique for CTC requires the patient to undergo a physical purging of the bowel before imaging. This is typically accomplished by one of two means, both of which involve the oral ingestion of cleansing agents. It should not be forgotten that patients find this process unpleasant. The bowel preparation contributes to the relatively poor compliance of individuals in the United States for colon screening programs (Brown et al. 1990; Weitzman 2001). As we shall discuss below, in response to this observation, there are efforts underway to modify the duress of the pre-exam bowel preparation.

In the so-called "wet prep," patients are asked to ingest approximately 4 L of a high-osmolality solution of polyethylene glycol electrolyte (PEG). The PEG is formulated to be nonabsorbable, and, hence, it draws fluid into the bowel, resulting in a physical purge. Ingestion begins the night before the procedure and typically lasts several hours. The nonabsorbed PEG solution mechanically flushes the bowel of its ingested contents effectively, and for this reason this agent has been used extensively in many centers as the standard preparation preceding abdominal surgery and lower endoscopy. However, in equal measure to its effectiveness at bowel cleansing, PEG causes patients to experience diarrhea. Patients frequently report that their discomfort and displeasure associated with the bowel prep equals if not exceeds their discomfort associated with the actual colon examination.

In contrast, the "dry" method relies on the cathartic action of pharmaceutical agents, including magnesium citrate, bisacoydl sodium, and phospha-soda, and is commercially available in a number of different preparations. Here, the patient ingests a combination of pills and suppositories starting the night before the exam, and the action of these agents promotes a physiologic purging of the bowel. The result is also an effective purging of the colon. As a result of this cathartic action, in addition to diarrhea, some patients report bowel cramping with the wet prep. However, in contrast to the wet prep, much less material must be ingested to effect complete cleansing.

To date, there is little published data evaluating the effect of preparation type on the diagnostic performance of CTC for detection of polyps. Macari et al. compared the amount of residual fluid present in the bowel using the wet vs dry techniques and observed that the dry method results in less retained fluid (Macari, Pedrosa, and Lavelle et al. 2001). The significance of this finding relates to the fact that unopacified bowel fluid and colonic polyps have essentially the same density. Therefore, by submerging polyps large amounts of unopacified fluid within the bowel may obscure polyps along the dependent surface of the distended colon. CTC is performed with both prone and supine acquisitions in part to address this problem. Fluid obscuring a lesion along one surface of the colon will be displaced on the other acquisition, in theory permitting clear evaluation. In principle, the use of the complementary prone and supine views in CTC is no different from the use of decubitus views of the colon in performing barium enemas. In CTC, both views are often critical to assessment due to variations in bowel distention in the two series. For example, in the sigmoid colon it is sometimes difficult to obtain adequate bowel distention and, as a result, optimal evaluation may only be possible on one series. Hence, if a large amount of fluid hinders evaluation of a region of colon in one view it may compromise the radiologist's ability to evaluate it with confidence. As a result, some centers avoid the wet preparation.

However, balanced against this potential disadvantage for the wet preparation is the fact that, if performed incompletely, the dry preparation can result in large amounts of retained fecal material. Desiccated fecal material can confound the radiologist's interpretation by mimicking the morphology of true polyps (Fletcher et al. 2000). Although a careful inspection of the cross-sectional density of a suspected lesion will usually reveal microbubbles of air in the case of a fecal pseudolesion, this inspection can be time consuming, especially if a large amount of retained material is present. Head-to-head comparison of the prep types is planned as part of an upcoming multicenter trial of CTC. Until a clear consensus emerges, it is advisable to educate patients as to the importance of the bowel preparation to promote compliance. Detailed evaluation of the colon is markedly diminished in the setting of an unprepped colon.

In addition to purgation cleansing of the bowel, diet modification has been employed to improve the quality of the preparation. In particular, it is common practice to advise patients to consume a low-residue diet for the 48 hours prior to exam. Foods containing large amounts of fiber, such as undercooked meats, fresh fruits, and vegetables, are to be avoided in favor of well-cooked items. This instruction derives from the extensive experience obtained with barium enemas and colonoscopy and is incorporated into the instructions of several commercially available dry preparations. There appears to be less of a requirement for diet modification with the wet prep, as the mechanical purging suffices to remove the ingested material from the colon. For both wet and dry preparations, patients should be encouraged to avoid ingesting solid food beginning the evening before the examination. On the morning of CTC, once the prep has essentially been completed, patients should be encouraged to adhere to a clear liquid diet until after the exam is finished. For patients with insulin-dependent diabetes, we follow the common practice of advising patients to reduce their morning insulin dose the morning of CTC; the examination should not precipitate problems with blood glucose control. In addition, as a courtesy and comfort measure, patients should be offered the chance to empty their bowel just prior to imaging. Several investigators have observed that on occasion the purging effects of both types of preps persist into the morning of the exam (Dachman et al. 1998; Fenlon and Ferrucci 1999). Some patients may be too embarrassed to mention this to the radiology staff at the scanner, but are nonetheless appreciative of the chance to relieve any pressure before air is insufflated into the colon. Immediately following image acquisition, all patients can return to their regular diet.

As a means to reduce the duress of pre-exam bowel preparation, several investigators have explored the possibility of replacing the purging process with a fecal tagging process, exploiting the fact that excellent oral-contrast agents exist for CT imaging. With this approach, patients are asked to ingest small aliquots of contrast with meals and snacks prior to imaging; this contrast material replaces the purging agents described above. The primary goal of this method is to thoroughly mark the ingested contents of the bowel so they appear distinct on subsequent CT images. Soft-tissue structures such as polyps and haustral folds do not absorb contrast material and so remain distinguishable because of their lower soft tissue density. Vining et al. (2001) reported on the use of barium agents ingested the morning of CTC in conjunction with a modified purging preparation. Callstrom et al. (2001) also reported on colonography using barium for fecal tagging but without the use of a purgative. Callstrom et al. (2001) observed that tagging of the ingested bowel contents is improved if the contrast regimen is ingested in divided doses starting 48 hours before imaging. In a limited cohort, they observed a sensitivity of 100% for detection of colonoscopically confirmed polyps >1 cm. Zalis and Hahn (2001) reported on the use of low-osmolar iodinated contrast agents, observing a statistically significant reader preference and an improved prep homogeneity when compared to barium agents.

It should be noted that with these techniques the 3D evaluation of the colon is limited by the presence of the opacified bowel contents and fluid. This endoluminal view of the colon mucosa is often useful as a means to evaluate indeterminate structures (Dachman et al. 1998; Beaulieu et al. 1999; McFarland et al. 2001).

Combining the use of tagging agents with a software-based removal of this material, Zalis and Hahn (2001) reported results of a process dubbed digital subtraction bowel cleansing. In this technique, specialized image processing algorithms remove the marked colon contents from the CT images as a postprocessing step, in effect cleaning the images rather than the patient. One potential advantage of this approach is that the 3D endoluminal evaluation of the colon is preserved for problem solving. In addition, the visually distracting tagged colon contents are removed from view during screening evaluation of the multiplanar images. In preliminary data obtained in a limited, enriched cohort of patients, two independent readers correctly identified all colonoscopy-confirmed polyps lower than 1 cm, suggesting performance comparable to standard CTC (Zalis et al. 2000; Zalis and Hahn 2001).

Investigators have also explored modifying the pre-exam bowel preparation for MR colonography. Lauenstein et al. (2001) recently employed a regimen of barium ingested prior to imaging to quench the signal of ingested colon contents.

Used in combination with a tap water enema and IV gadolinium contrast, the barium admixture renders the ingested colon material dark against a background of brightly enhancing colonic mucosa. In a limited cohort, these investigators observed an overall sensitivity of 91% for detection of colonoscopically confirmed polyps.

The results of all these studies are encouraging, but at the time of this writing no large trial has yet been conducted that conclusively demonstrates the effectiveness of these approaches in a screening population. Hence, these preliminary data point toward a promising avenue of research, but they require further validation before being accepted as guidance for standard practice.

Conclusion

In addition to possible cost savings and time efficiency, the usefulness of CTC lies in part with its potential to improve the patient's experience before and during colon examination. By educating patients to develop an appropriate set of expectations about the exam, the radiology staff can help reduce the anxiety experienced by many patients approaching colon evaluation. The importance of these matters cannot be overstated. Good patient preparation is essential for the acquisition of high-quality CTC images and requires active compliance on the part of the patient. Several lines of research are being pursued to reduce the duress of the pre-exam cleansing, and, in the near future, a combination of fecal tagging and electronic cleansing may replace the current regimen.

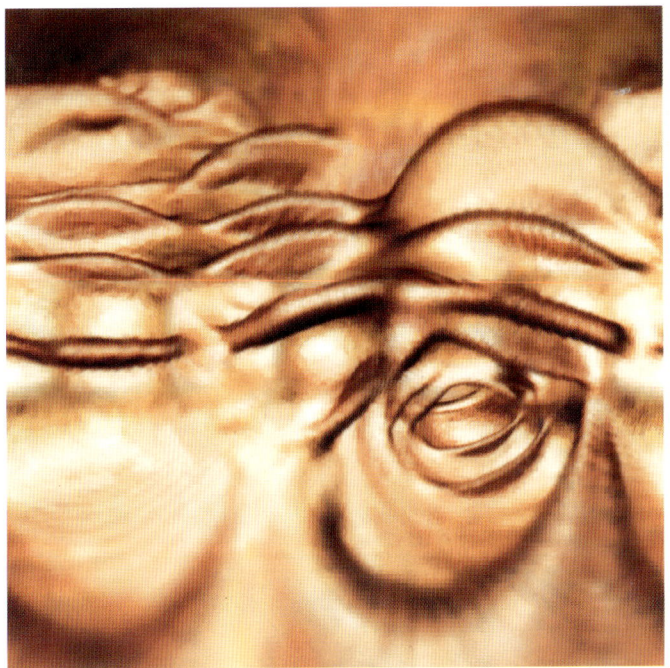

A

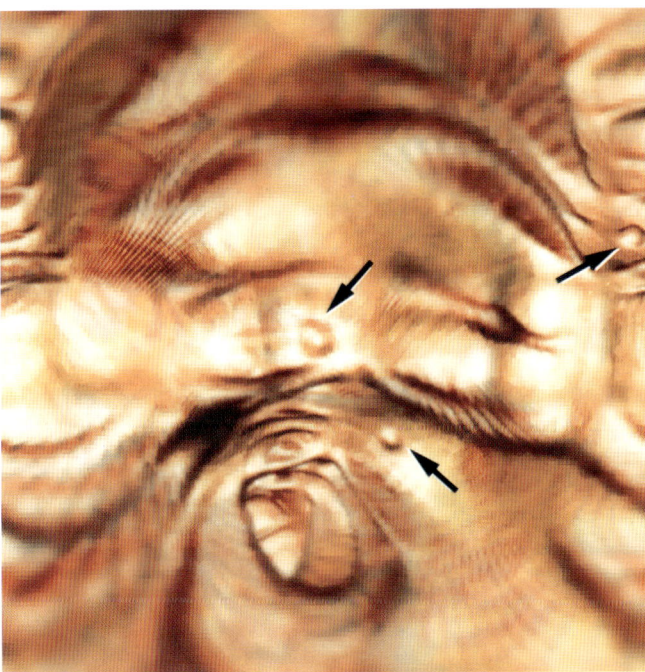

B

FIGURE 6.6. Mercator projection virtual endoscopy. (**A**) A total of 18 camera renderings have been knitted together to depict normal colon morphology. (**B**) Mercator projection from another segment of colon shows several polyps (arrows).

FIGURE 6.7. Virtual gross pathology. Reformatted tomograms along the colon centerline were used to create a new 3D volume, which was subsequently flattened and volume rendered. Enlargements of segments of the overall colon show haustral fold anatomy and a 1.5 cm polypoid lesion (lipoma, arrow).

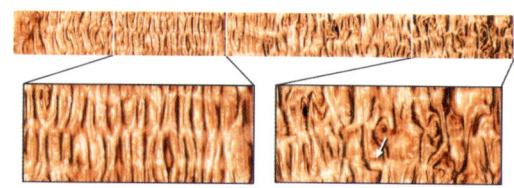

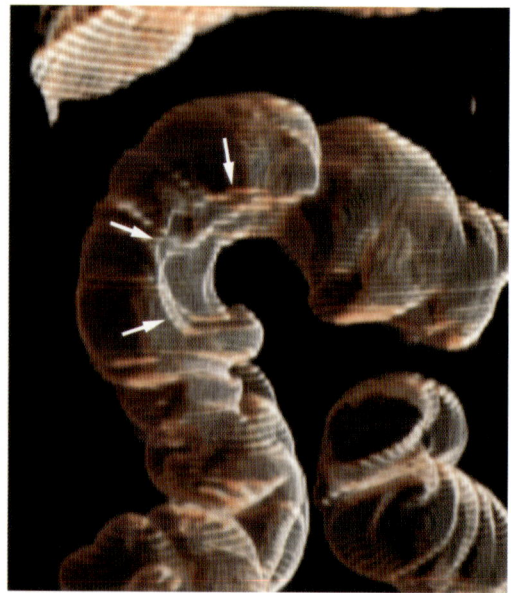

FIGURE 6.8. Tissue transition projection. 3D volume rendering of the colon in the region of the hepatic flexure shows a filling defect along the inner aspect of the flexure due to a 2.5 cm carcinoma (arrows).

FIGURE 8.1. Conceptual diagram of colonic surface shape showing haustral folds (green), polyps (orange-red), and normal colonic surface between folds (yellow). A polyp on a fold (small arrow) and one between folds (large arrow) are shown. Polyps can be distinguished from folds and normal colonic mucosa by their distinctive shapes. (Used with permission from Summers 2000b.)

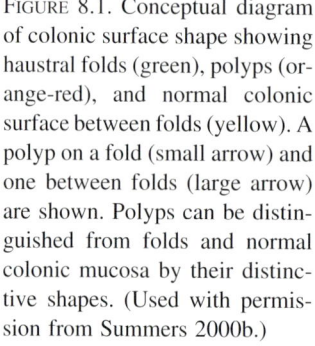

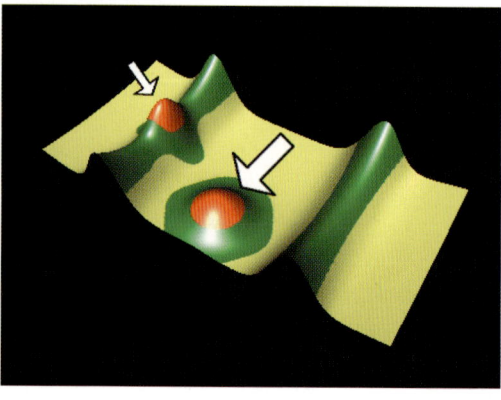

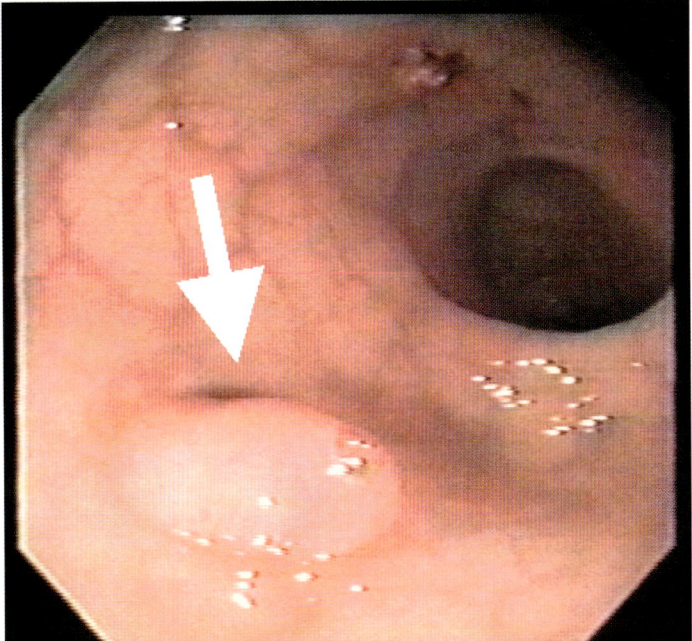

A

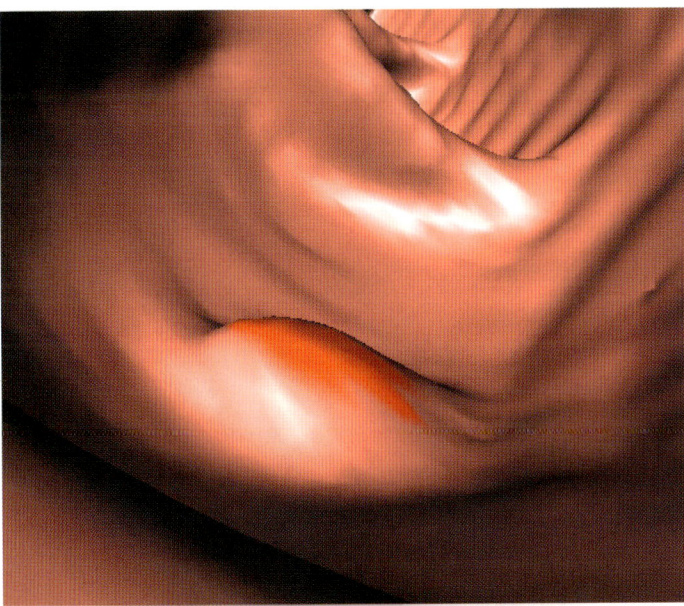

B

FIGURE 8.2. Examples of three polyps (arrows) measuring 1 to 1.5 cm in size. (**A,C,E**) Conventional colonoscopy and (**B,D,F**) corresponding CT colonography perspective renderings. In (**B,D,F**), red coloring indicates portion of polyps detected by computer-assisted detection algorithm. Note the absence of false positive diagnoses on folds and normal colonic mucosa. (Used with permission from Summers et al. 2001c.)

Continues on next page

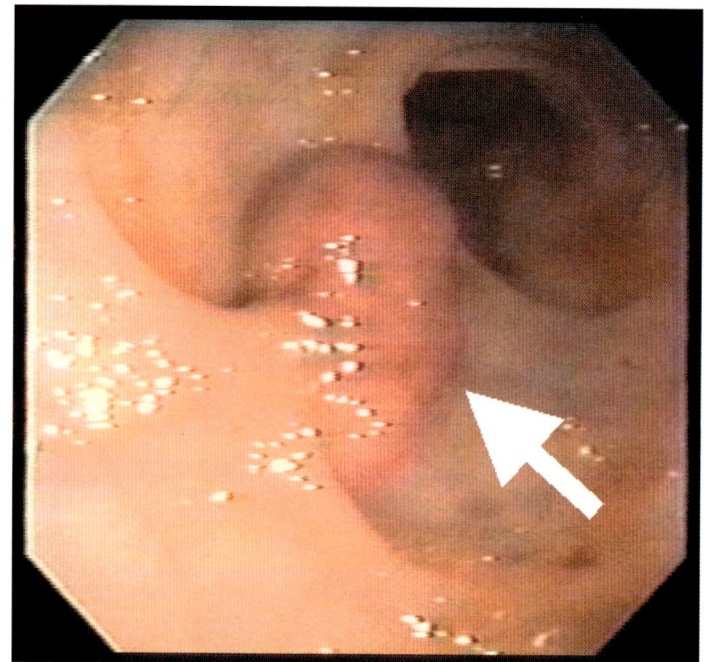

C

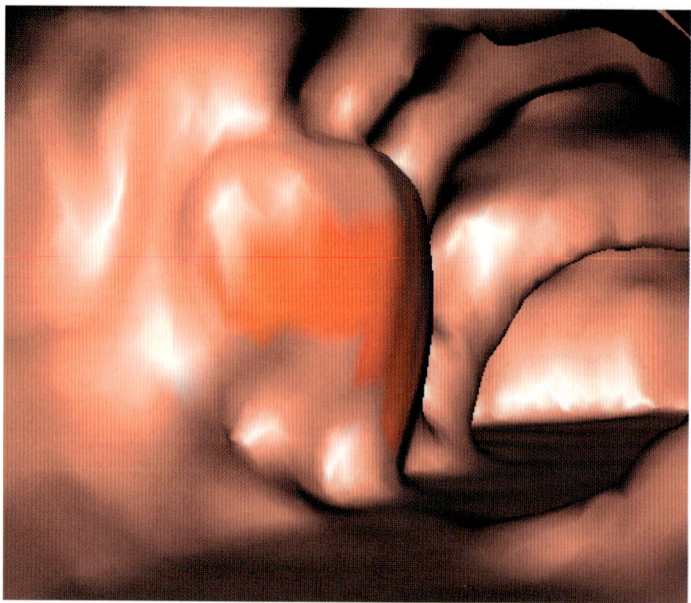

D

FIGURE 8.2. (*Continued*)

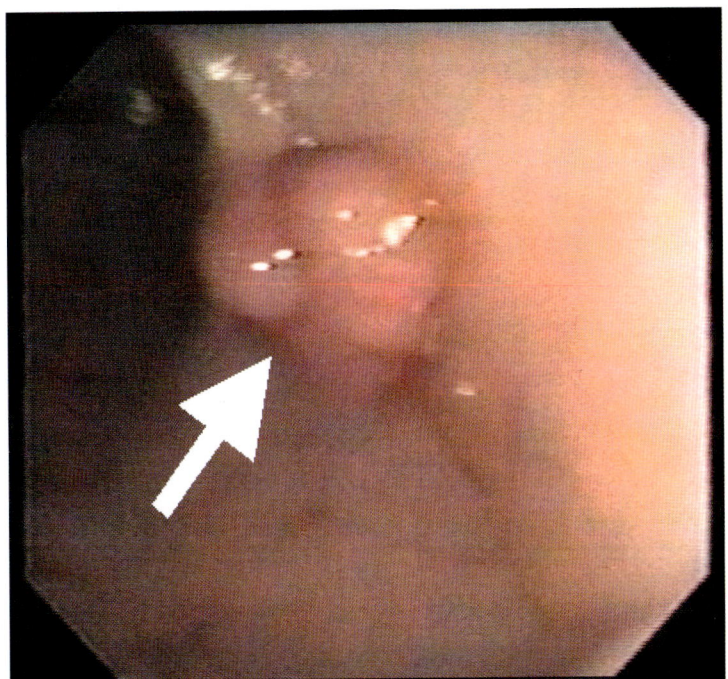

E

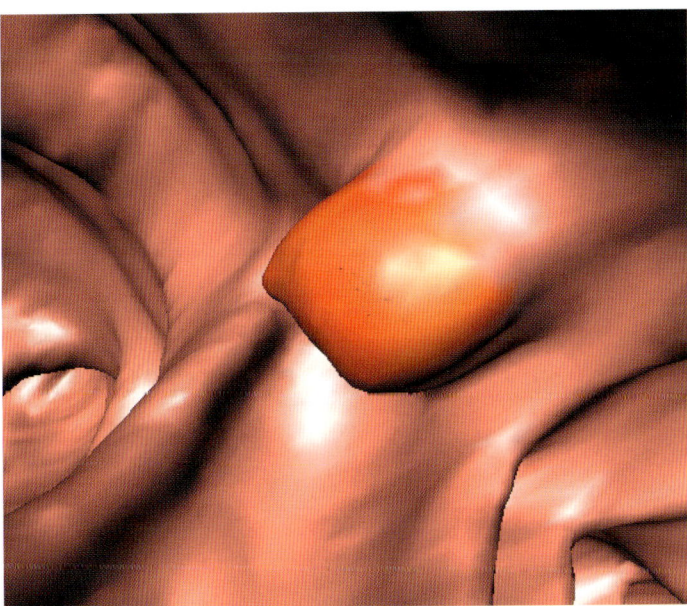

F

FIGURE 8.2. (*Continued*)

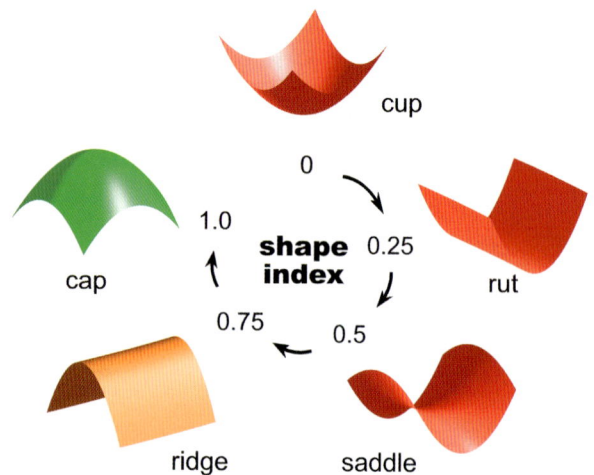

cup

0

shape 0.25
index

1.0

cap

ridge 0.75 0.5

rut

saddle

FIGURE 8.4. Relationship between the volumetric shape index values and shape classes. Polyps tend to appear as bulbous, cap-like structures adhering to the colonic wall, and thus have a shape index value close to 1. Folds appear as elongated, ridge-like structures, and have a shape index value of approximately 0.75. The colonic wall appears as a large, nearly flat, cup-like structure, and has a shape index value of close of 0. By coloring voxels that have shape index values corresponding to the cap, saddle to ridge, and the other classes by green, pink, and brown, respectively, one can distinguish these structures clearly (see Fig. 8.5). (Used with permission from Yoshida, Masutani, and MacEneaney et al. 2002.)

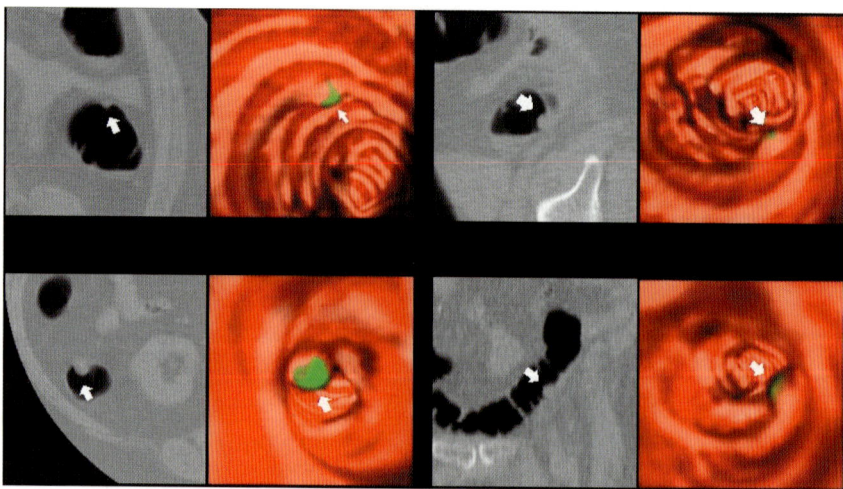

FIGURE 8.5. Effect of the volumetric shape index in differentiation among polyps, folds, and the colonic wall. In each pair of images, an axial or coronal CT image that contains a polyp indicated by arrow is shown on the left and its 3D endoscopic views by perspective volume rendering is shown on the right: (**A**) 6 mm polyp in sigmoid, (**B**) 9 mm polyp in sigmoid, (**C**) 8 mm polyp in sigmoid, (**D**) 9 mm polyp in sigmoid. With the coloring scheme shown in Fig 8.4, polyps, folds, and the colonic wall are clearly separated, and the polyps are easily distinguishable from other structures. (Used with permission from Yoshida, Nappi, and MacEneaney et al. 2002; Yoshida and Nappi 2001.)

6

Advanced 3D Display Methods

Christopher F. Beaulieu, David S. Paik, Sandy Napel,
and R. Brooke Jeffrey, Jr.

With conventional 2D computed tomography (CT) sections, polyps may be difficult to detect and, conversely, normal structures such as haustra may appear polypoid and be mistaken as pathology. This provides the rationale for 3D displays such as virtual endoscopy, which depicts more intuitively the topographical features of the colon. At the same time, 3D displays in and of themselves are insufficient to fully characterize a suspected polyp because CT attenuation values provide clues as to whether an area represents soft tissue or fat, or if the area contains gas as often found in foci of retained stool.

Although it is widely accepted that both 2D and 3D displays reveal important features for polyp diagnosis (Dachman et al. 1998), there is not yet a consensus on which 2D or 3D viewing modes provide for the most accurate and efficient diagnosis. Moreover, advances in image processing and computer graphics have led to a multitude of advanced 3D displays that go beyond "conventional" virtual endoscopy, defined as the 3D view created when a *single* virtual camera is positioned inside the colonic lumen.

This chapter describes the concepts and potential advantages of these advanced viewing modes. We begin with a brief description of virtual camera navigation and perspective rendering principles, then illustrate several advanced viewing modes, based both on "optical" unraveling of the colon and on "tomographic" unraveling.

Navigation and Perspective Rendering

A CT colonographic dataset is a 3D array of voxels, each of which is characterized by its spatial (x,y,z) location and attenuation value. Because the array does not possess a priori information as to which voxels belong to the colon, some process of identifying the colon within the array is necessary before virtual endoscopic viewing becomes possible. An experienced observer can perform this localization visually, relying on anatomic knowledge and attenuation cues. With appropriate computer software, one can also select a local area within the colon to serve as a position for the virtual camera. In addition, one can point the camera in a chosen direction toward the colonic wall or along the lumen. Once positioned and oriented, 3D graphics software is used to render the colonic surface with a rendering algorithm such as shaded surface display (Lorensen and Cline 1987) or volume rendering (Johnson et al. 1996; Rubin et al. 1996). While a detailed description of 3D rendering algorithms is beyond the scope of this chapter, it is useful to further discuss navigation through the volume and virtual camera field of view (FOV).

Once a virtual camera is positioned at a particular voxel, moving the camera's position to another voxel will result in a new 3D rendering of the surface. Sequential movement of the camera along the colon amounts to navigating its course, wherein the goal is to view the surface in an animated, fly-through format. Various research groups have developed software packages that make this process a semiautomatic, preprocessing step (Paik et al. 1998; Reed and Johnson 1997; Samara et al. 1999; Lorensen et al. 1995). While specific implementations differ, most of these algorithms perform an initial segmentation of the air–attenuation colon voxels by nearest-neighbor connectivity (Cline et al. 1987), followed by a scheme to compute a path along the axis of the colon along which to drive the virtual camera (Fig 6.1). Designing a program to compute a path that is *centered* in the colon is difficult, but the utility of a central axis path is much higher than that of a shortest-distance path. One advantage of a central axis path is that it centers the viewing *frustum* (the conical "visual field") of the virtual camera, whereas the shortest-distance path tends to hug the colon walls, especially around curvatures. This latter effect is not only visually unappealing, but may reduce the amount of colon surface actually depicted during an endoscopic fly-through. Another advantage of generating a central axis path is that the path points serve as the basis for further image processing and analytic tools. For example, path points may serve as the axis of rotation for generation of tomograms that can be instantaneously perpendic-ular or parallel to the path. These reformatted tomograms can be used for image viewing directly or used to create a new volumetric dataset for 3D rendering, as discussed later.

Some newer commercial software packages enable flight through the colon without explicit computation of a central axis path. In some cases, these programs employ collision detection schemes to avoid too close an approach of the virtual camera to the colon wall.

By tradition, 3D rendering has used parallel rays cast through the imaging data to generate an image. With this approach, moving closer to the data amounts to magnification, at the expense of the orientation of the viewer. With *perspective* graphics, nonparallel, divergent rendering rays are used. This allows the viewer to more closely approach the object without losing orientation and enables effective viewing of the dataset from within, as opposed to being limited to external viewpoints. The *viewing frustum* of the camera is the pyramidal area of space within view and the *solid angle* of an object about a point is defined as the surface area of a unit sphere centered on the point that is subtended by the object. By varying the degree of divergence of the rendering rays, perspective virtual cameras effectively change their viewing frustum, or FOV, analogous to switch-

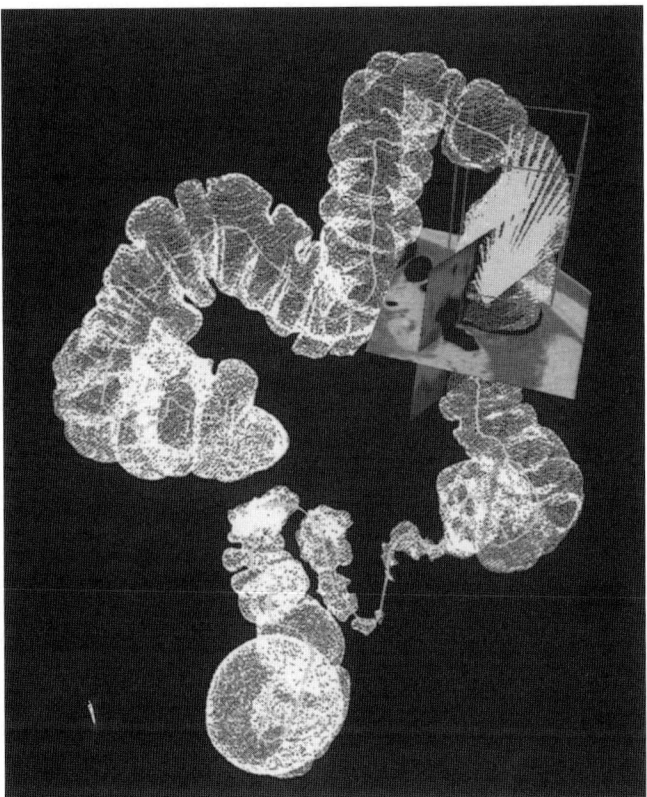

FIGURE 6.1. Navigation and centerline path. The air-containing colon from a 3D CTC dataset has been segmented, as represented by the point cloud. A computer algorithm has been used to create a centerline path, and the centerline is used to position and orient the virtual camera, as illustrated by the bounding box and rays cast along the colon.

ing lenses on a conventional camera. A 60° FOV virtual camera displays only 8.3% of the solid angle available for viewing, thereby missing over 90% of the available solid angle. Increasing the FOV to 180° only visualizes half of the surrounding solid angle. By using two diametrically opposed 180° FOV cameras, the entire solid angle can be visualized. However, wide-angle lenses suffer increasing geometric distortion with increasing FOV, thereby limiting useful FOV to 80° to 100° for a single camera (Fig 6.2) (Paik et al. 2000).

Depending on the specifics of the computer graphics system used (Wax et al. 2001), the percentage surface visual-ization for both single-direction and bidirectional 60° FOV cameras may be relatively low (approximately 75% of the total surface [Paik et al. 2000]) and therefore lead to missed polyps because portions of the surface are not displayed to the observer (Beaulieu et al. 1999).

Another limitation of virtual colonoscopy using a reasonably nondistorting FOV is that the virtual camera must constantly be panned to maximize the per-

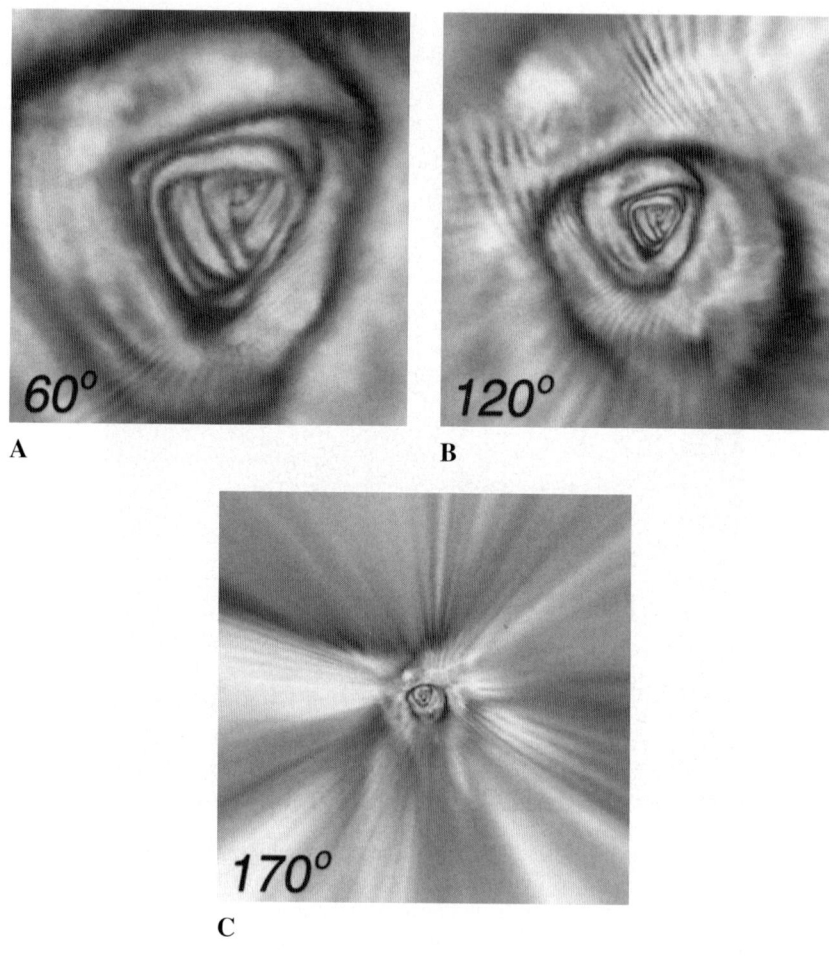

FIGURE 6.2. Single-camera virtual endoscopy. At a FOV of 60° (**A**), haustral folds project into the lumen, limiting visibility. At 120° (**B**) and 170° (**C**), perspective distortion occurs, effectively limiting the upper limit on camera FOV to around 100°. (Used with permission from Paik et al. 2000.)

centage of total solid angle visualized. This panning must also be done to visualize in between haustral folds, which tend to limit the view of the colonic surface by occluding the view behind them (Fig 6.3). In fiber optic colonoscopy, the tip of the colonoscope can be manually diverted to look in between each fold. However, to do this in virtual colonoscopy requires hardware and software capable of real-time rendering as well as considerable operator time and skill.

The limitations in surface viewing and perspective distortion were the main motivations for developing alternative approaches to virtual endoscopy that utilize multiple, midrange (~60°) FOV virtual cameras with different orientations to display as much as the local colon topology as possible.

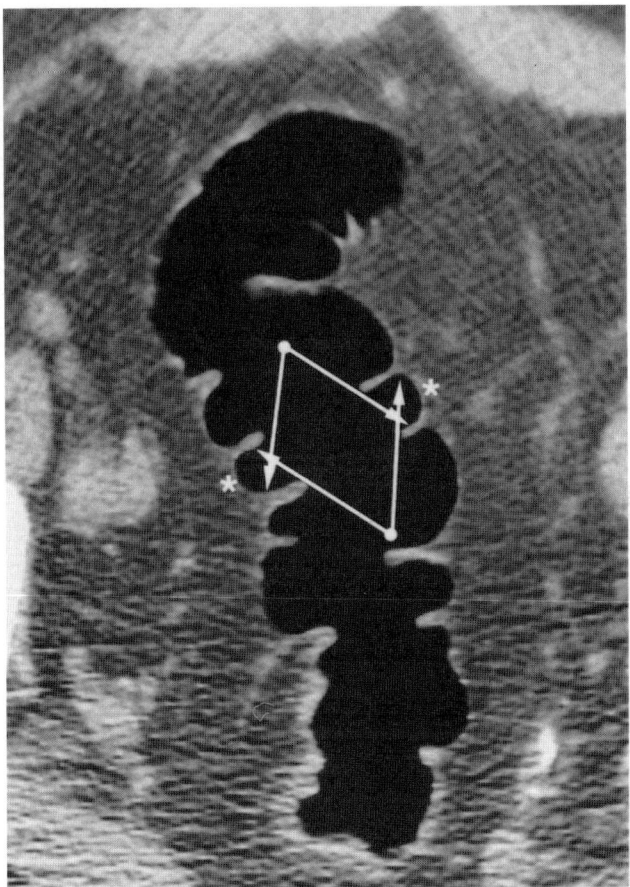

FIGURE 6.3. Limited visibility of single-camera virtual endoscopy. Segment of colon depicted on axial CT image with camera position and viewpoints depicted by arrows. Areas in between haustral folds (*) may not be fully visualized due to limitations in camera FOV and viewing angle. (Used with permission from Paik et al. 2000.)

Panoramic Viewing and Map Projections

An optimal viewing method for virtual colonoscopy would be one that includes a minimally distorting graphics projection while visualizing the entire surface of the colon. One fairly obvious extension of single-camera virtual colonoscopy is to create a montage view using multiple cameras pointed in different directions. Figure 6.4 illustrates one such view, created when a single central camera (60° FOV) is surrounded by eight additional cameras oriented at angles of 60° with respect to the centerline path (Sheikh et al. 1998). In the extreme condition which the peripheral cameras are oriented at 90° to the path, one obtains a panoramic view of a strip of surrounding colon (Beaulieu et al. 1999). An illustration of the viewing directions is shown in Figure 6.5A and an example of a panoramic colon

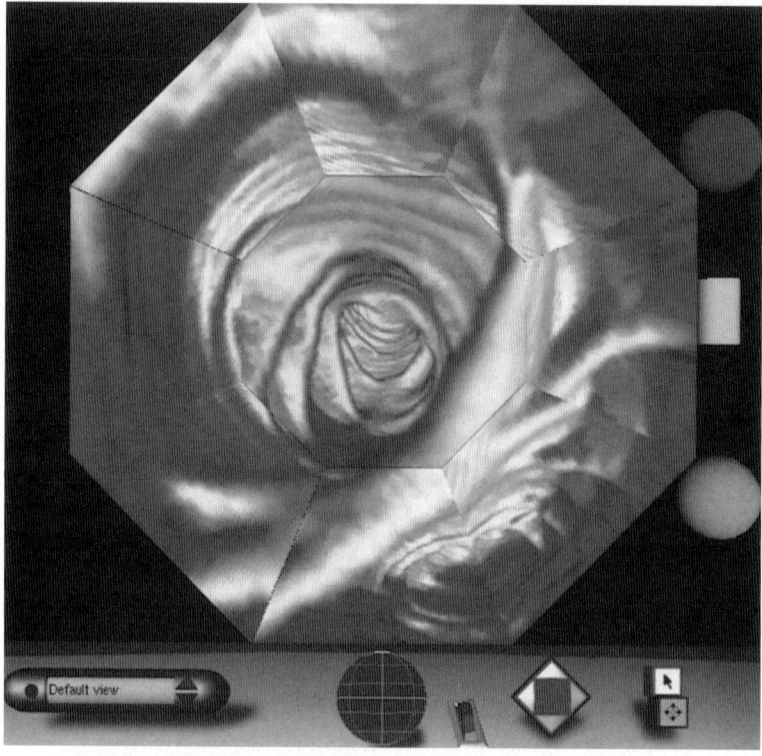

FIGURE 6.4. Virtual cockpit. A total of nine 60° cameras were used to create a wide-angle viewing method without perspective distortion.

view is shown in Figure 6.5B. To view the entire colon, one creates a movie of sequential panoramic views from each path point. The advantage of the panoramic projection is that it maximizes visibility of the colon in between haustral folds. The main disadvantage is that it is difficult to anticipate lesions that may be coming into the viewing area, as the view only extends over ~3 to 4 cm along the path at any given path viewing point.

Conceptually, translating the colon (or a spherical viewing area centered at any point in the lumen) onto a flat viewing surface is similar to that faced by mapmakers desiring to visualize the surface of a sphere (e.g., the Earth) mapped onto a flat surface. Elegant solutions to this problem were initially conceived by Ptolemy in the second century AD.

There are three major classes of map projections: planar, cylindrical, and conic (Paik et al. 2000; Robinson 1995; Snyder 1993). These are the projections of the surface of the globe from a single point inside the globe onto various surfaces that are easily transformed to the plane. Conic, cylindrical, and planar projections result from projecting onto a cone, cylinder, or plane, respectively. The 360° panoramic cameras used to photograph landscapes are best modeled by cylindrical projections. These cameras capture 360° of landscape surrounding the

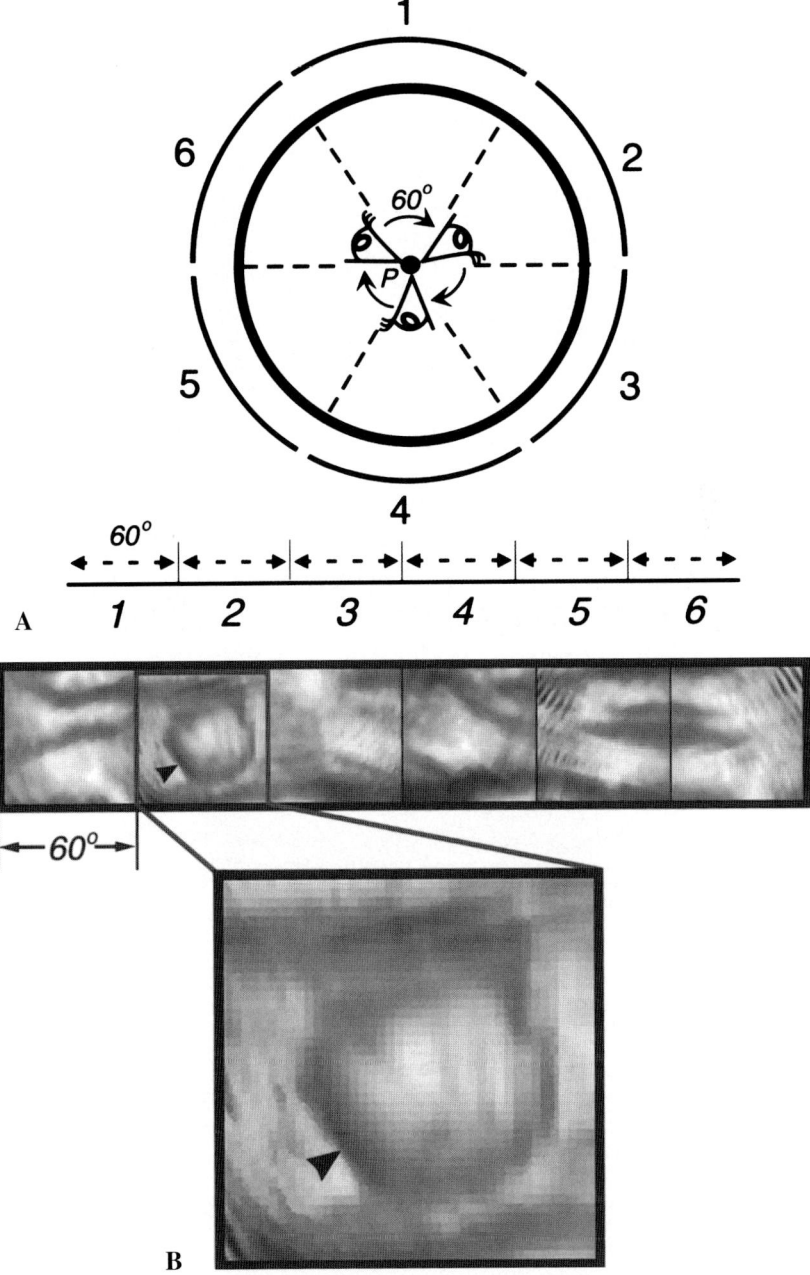

FIGURE 6.5. Panoramic virtual endoscopy. (**A**) Schematic of virtual camera viewing directions. Six cameras are oriented perpendicular to the centerline path, at 60° angles with respect to one another, creating six images of the surrounding colon wall, illustrated by segments 1–6. When knitted together, a circumferential view of the colon is created, as illustrated in the lower portion of the figure. (**B**) Example of panoramic endoscopy with six virtual cameras. Enlargement from the upper panel shows a 10-mm polyp (arrowhead). (Used with permission from Beaulieu et al. 1999.)

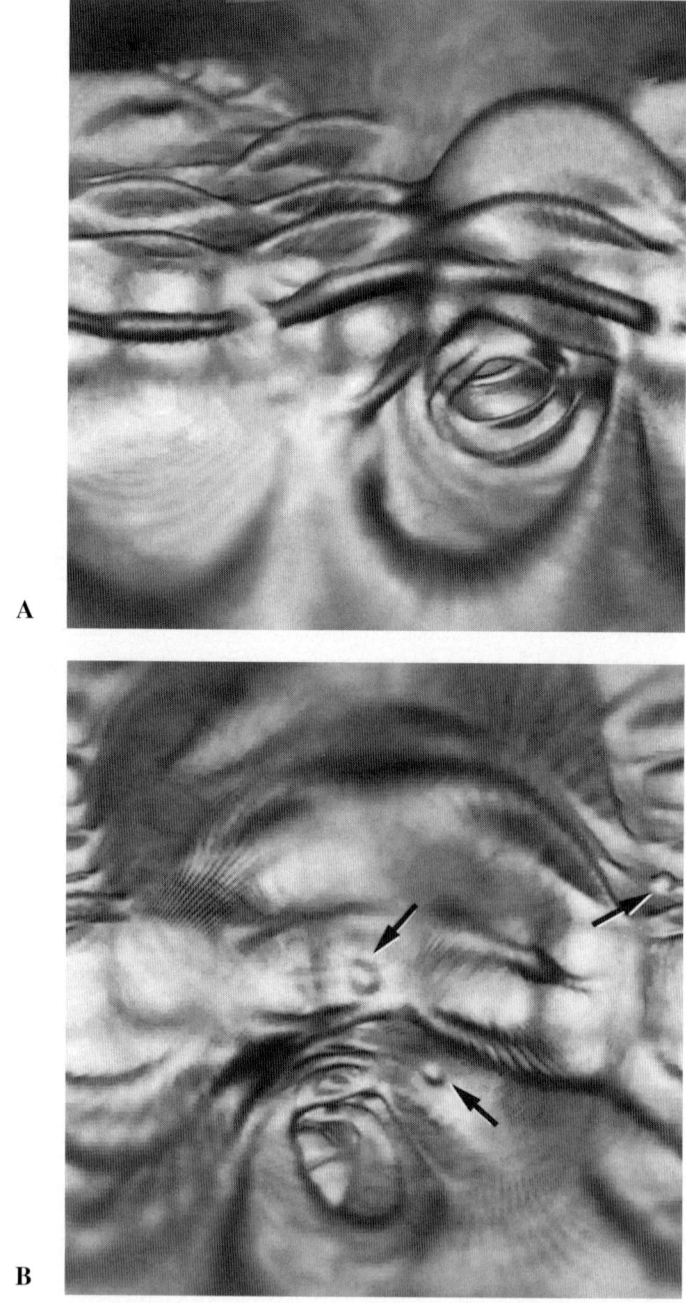

FIGURE 6.6. Mercator projection virtual endoscopy. (**A**) A total of 18 camera renderings have been knitted together to depict normal colon morphology. (**B**) Mercator projection from another segment of colon shows several polyps (arrows). (See color insert)

camera by focusing light onto a cylindrical piece of film as the aperture is rotated. The simplest type of cylindrical projection is the *equirectangular projection*, where lines of latitude and longitude are mapped directly to an equirectangular grid. Another well-known cylindrical projection is the *Mercator projection*, which projects the surface of the globe onto a tangent cylinder from the center of the globe (Fig 6.6; see color insert). Attractive features of the Mercator projection are preservation of aspect ratio across the field (i.e., like stereographic projection, spheres are projected as circles) and that all objects are displayed with minimum distortion at the equator (horizontal line bisecting the image). However, the poles of the globe are mapped infinitely far away on the map.

Both panoramic and map projections have been compared with axial CT and single-camera virtual endoscopy by our group (Paik et al. 2000; Beaulieu et al. 1999). In these blinded reader trials using simulated polyps, we found that the 3D modes led to higher detection sensitivity than the axial, 2D mode.

Tomographic Colon Unraveling

Whereas the map projections described above utilize a number of virtual camera views knitted together to increase the amount of colon surface visualized, it is also possible to straighten and flatten the colon by reformation of the axial CT data. In its simplest form, tomograms perpendicular to the central axis of the colon are generated at intervals along the path. These reformatted tomograms are then stacked together into a new volume. The new volume may be visualized as cylindrical or further flattened into a view that appears similar to the colon at gross pathologic examination, leading to the term "virtual gross pathology" (Fig 6.7; see color insert). A significant limitation of reformations instantaneously perpendicular to the central colon path is that under- or oversampling of the wall voxels may occur in flexures, leading to skipped areas of the wall or duplication

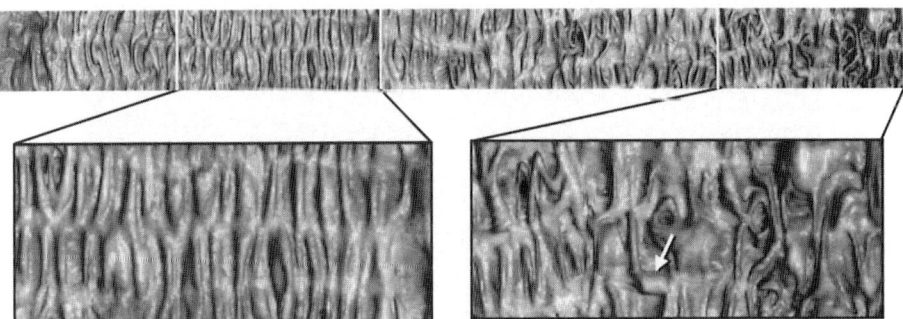

FIGURE 6.7. Virtual gross pathology. Reformatted tomograms along the colon centerline were used to create a new 3D volume, which was subsequently flattened and volume rendered. Enlargements of segments of the overall colon show haustral fold anatomy and a 1.5-cm polypoid lesion (lipoma, arrow). (See color insert)

of abnormalities. One approach to minimizing such distortions is to modify the reformatted tomograms according to colonic curvature, resulting in more uniform sampling of the colon wall (Wang et al. 1998; Dave et al. 1999).

While there is strong appeal in viewing the colon as a single or small number of virtual gross pathologic views, at this point there have not been systematic studies of the efficacy of this viewing mode relative to axial CT sections or more conventional 3D viewing modes.

Other Volume-Rendering Methods

In addition to the virtual camera-based approaches and extensions described above, there are a multitude of methods for viewing the colonic surface with

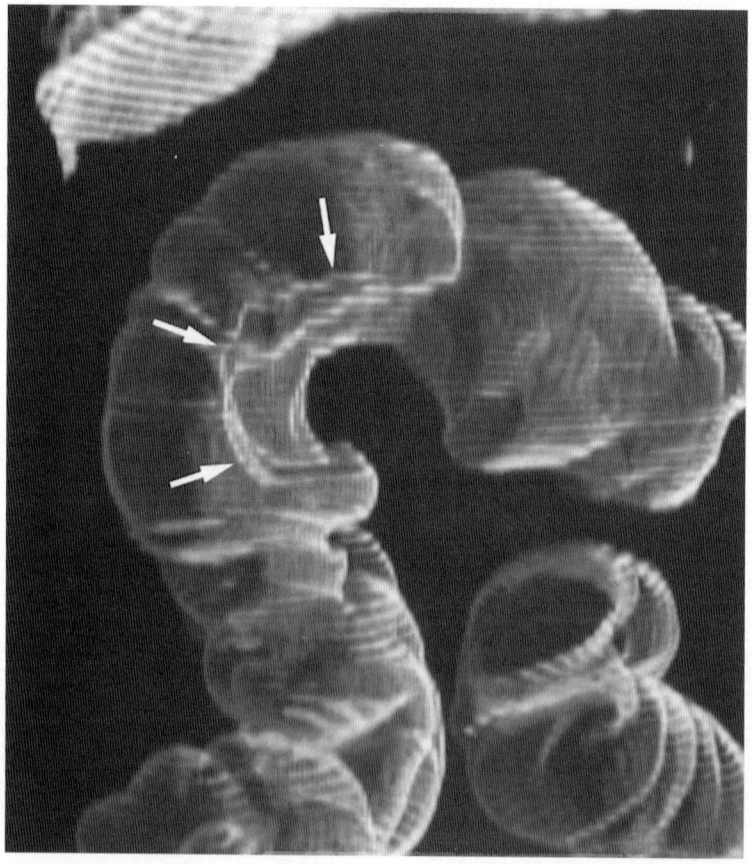

FIGURE 6.8. Tissue transition projection. 3D volume rendering of the colon in the region of the hepatic flexure shows a filling defect along the inner aspect of the flexure due to a 2.5-cm carcinoma (arrows). (See color insert)

computer graphics. In one method, a colonic centerline is created, and then the colon is split along this axis into halves, allowing a "clamshell" view of the inner surface. In another method, the voxels along the colon wall are rendered selectively (Fig 6.8; see color insert), simulating a double-contrast barium enema (Rogalla et al. 2000).

Finally, a fairly simple method of viewing the colon surface is to render a slab of the volumetric dataset (Fig 6.9), enabling a 3D view of polyps but avoiding the necessity of actually navigating through the colon (McFarland et al. 2001). In this method, one constructs a series of overlapping slabs with axial, coronal, or sagittal orientation and views them as "sliding slabs" analogous to sliding thin-slab maximum-intensity projection displays (Napel et al. 1993).

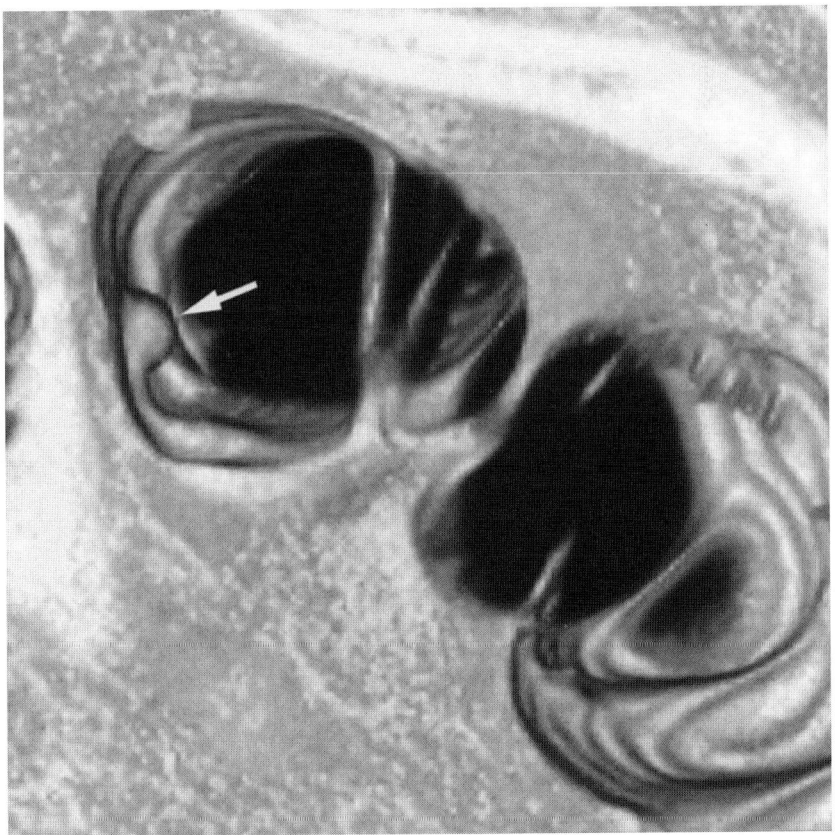

FIGURE 6.9. Slab volume rendering. Localized area in the splenic flexure rendered as a 20-mm-thick, volume-rendered slab, shows 10-mm polyp along the colon surface. This type of display combines the positive attributes of 2D and 3D display and does not require generation of a colon centerline. For complete colon viewing, a series of overlapping slabs is viewed in movie format.

Future Developments

Virtual endoscopic viewing has been shown to be an important adjunct to viewing of 2D sections in interpretation of CT colonography (CTC), and some would argue that the initial mode of data review should be with 3D fly-through visualization. In this chapter, we illustrated an array of more advanced computer graphics methods that increase the amount of colon surface viewed compared with single-camera endoscopy. These methods should further enhance the task of polyp detection on 3D images. The optimal clinical application for CTC is to achieve a high-sensitivity, high-specificity exam that can be interpreted in a time frame appropriate for an inexpensive, screening study. Despite the advanced computer graphics techniques described here, efficiency issues have not been seriously addressed. In this regard, some research labs have turned to computer-aided detection (CAD) for primary evaluation of the colon, followed by radiologist viewing of suspicious areas as defined by the computer (Paik et al. 1999; Summers et al. 2000b, 2001). If highly sensitive polyp-finding algorithms can be developed, the time spent examining a large amount of normal colon wall can be minimized, thereby maximizing efficiency. With the appropriate combination of sensitivity, specificity, and CAD-directed efficiency, CTC has a promising future for widespread acceptance.

7

MR Colonography

Thomas C. Lauenstein and Jörg F. Debatin

Colorectal cancer (CRC) remains the second leading cause of cancer mortality in western countries. Approximately 6% of the population will develop CRC during their lifetime (Neuhaus 1999). The majority of colon cancers develop from nonmalignant adenomas or polyps (O'Brien et al. 1990). Thus, cancer screening programs targeting precancerous polyps with subsequent endoscopic polypectomy could significantly reduce the incidence and hence the mortality of CRC.

Insufficient diagnostic accuracy and/or poor patient acceptance characterize most available colorectal screening modalities, including testing for occult fecal blood, conventional colonoscopy, or double-contrast barium enema (Frommer 1998; Ahlquist et al. 1993). Virtual colonography (VC), based on 3D computed tomography (CT) or magnetic resonance (MR) data sets has been found to be highly sensitive for detecting clinically relevant colorectal polyps exceeding 8 mm (Fenlon et al. 1999; Pappalardo et al. 2000). Although CT colonography (CTC) has considerable advantages regarding spatial resolution, examination cost, and scanner availability, the lack of harmful side effects, including ionizing radiation in addition to an unsurpassed soft-tissue contrast potential, render MR imaging (MRI) attractive as an alternative imaging modality for colorectal screening.

MR Colonography: Technique

Currently, two techniques are being evaluated for MR colonography (MRC). Based on the signal within the colonic lumen, these techniques can be differentiated as "bright-lumen" and "dark-lumen" MRC.

Bright-Lumen MRC

Similar to contrast-enhanced 3D MR angiography, MRC is based on the principles of ultrafast, T_1-weighted 3D gradient echo (GRE) acquisitions collected within the confines of a single breath hold (Luboldt et al. 1997). This requires the use of an MR scanner equipped with high-performance gradients. To permit homogeneous signal transmission and reception over the entire colon with high CNR values, a combination of phased-array surface coils should be used. The size of the coil must permit coverage of the entire colon. Because colonic lesions often cannot be differentiated from stool, the patient has to undergo bowel cleansing in a manner similar to that required for conventional colonoscopy. Prior to the examination, the patient should be screened for contraindications to MRI such as severe claustrophobia, presence of metallic implants in critical regions such as the eyes, spinal cord, or brain, or cardiac pacemakers. The presence of hip prostheses, normally not regarded a contraindication to MRI, impedes a complete analysis of the rectum and sigmoid colon. Therefore, patients with hip prostheses should also not be examined by MRC.

After placement of a rectal enema tube, the colon is filled with the patient in the prone position using 2500 to 3000 mL of a water-based enema, spiked with paramagnetic contrast (1:100). The enema is administered using 100 to 150 cm of hydrostatic pressure. To reduce bowel motion and alleviate colonic spasm, the use of intravenously administered spasmolytic agents (e.g., scopolamine or glucagon) prior to and during the bowel filling is helpful. In contrast to conventional colonoscopy, neither sedatives nor analgesic agents are routinely administered. To ensure safe and optimal bowel filling and distension, the filling process is monitored with a non-slice–select 2D acquisition, collecting one image every 3 seconds (Fig 7.1). Once the enema has reached the cecum, a 3D dataset of the abdomen encompassing the entire colon is collected. To compensate for the presence of residual air exhibiting "filling defects" similar to polyps within the colonic lumen, 3D datasets are collected in both the prone and supine patient positions (Fig 7.2). The enema bag is then placed on the floor to facilitate emptying of the colon, and the patient is removed from the scanner.

The acquired 3D MR datasets consist of coronal sections, ranging in thickness between 1.5 and 2 mm. The sequence is based on the use of short repetition (TR 1.6 to 3.8 ms) and echo times (0.6 to 1.6 ms). The achievable minimum TR should be shorter than 5 ms; otherwise, the acquisition of a 3D dataset cannot be collected within the confines of a single breath hold. In conjunction with a field of view of 400 × 400 mm and an imaging matrix of 460 × 512, the spatial resolution includes an interpolated voxel size of approximately 1 × 1 × 1.6 mm.

On the 3D GRE datasets, only the colonic lumen containing the enema is bright, whereas all other tissues remain low in signal intensity (Fig 7.3). The resulting contrast between the colonic lumen and surrounding structures is the basis for subsequent virtual colonographic viewing (Fig 7.4). The MRC protocol can be further amplified by the acquisition of 2D gradient-echo data sets following the intravenous (IV) application of a gadolinium-containing contrast compound. This permits a more comprehensive assessment of parenchymal abdominal organs and enhances the ability to detect hepatic metastases.

Bright-lumen MRC can be completed within 20 minutes, including the time for patient positioning, image planning, and data acquisition. The 3D datasets are subsequently postprocessed using commercially available software and hardware.

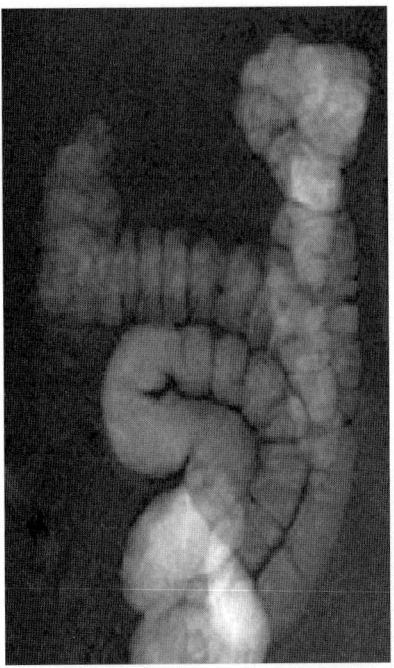
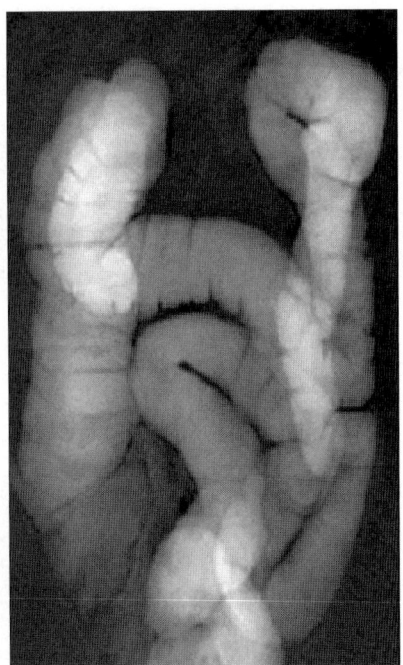

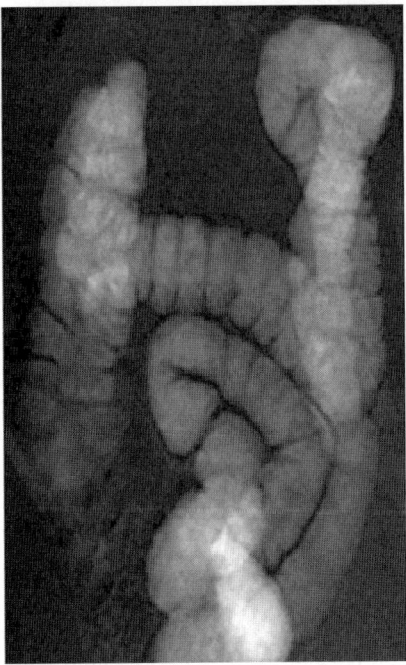

FIGURE 7.1. Colonic filling is monitored with a non-slice–select 2D acquisition collecting one image every 3 seconds. The far-right image demonstrates that enema has reached the cecum.

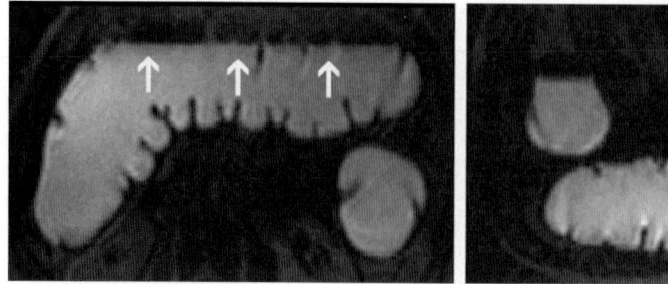

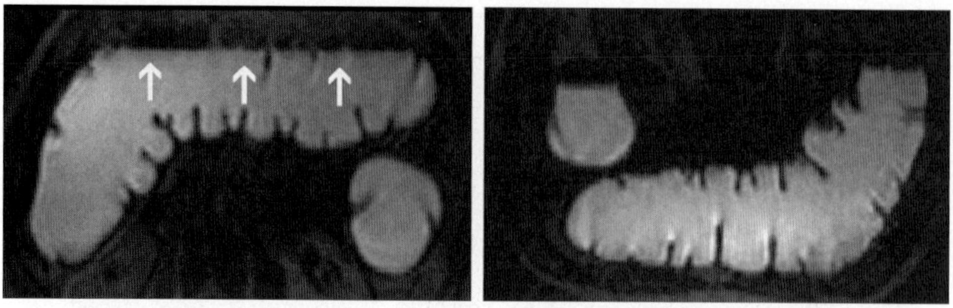

FIGURE 7.2. To compensate for the presence of residual air (left), the 3D dataset is collected once in the prone and a second time in the supine position. Residual air alters its position (right) due to gravity.

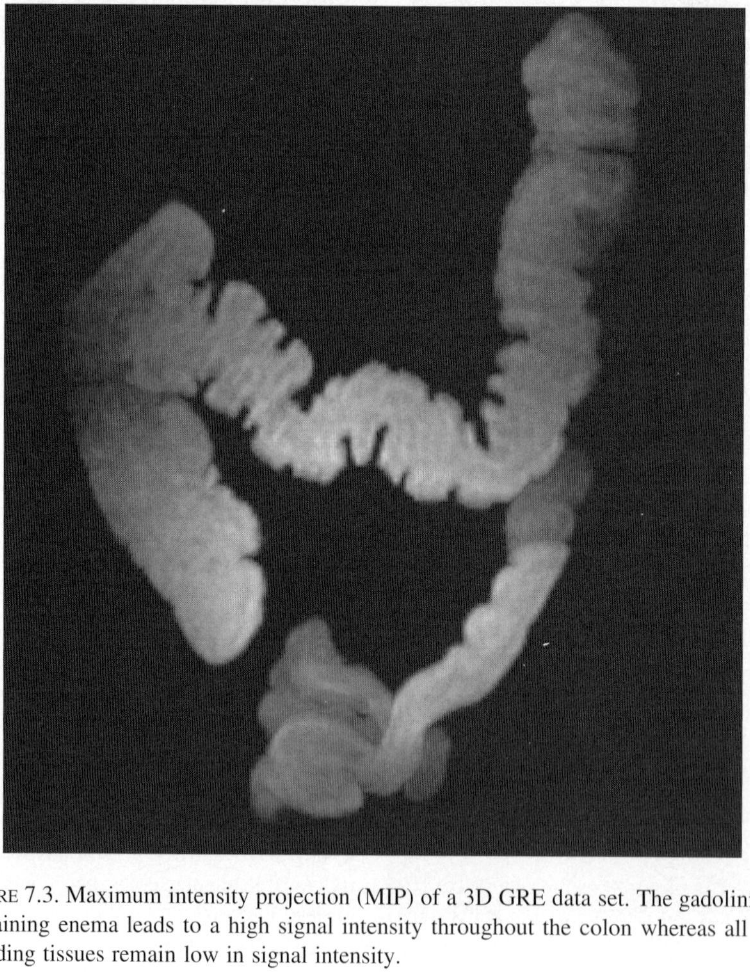

FIGURE 7.3. Maximum intensity projection (MIP) of a 3D GRE data set. The gadolinium-containing enema leads to a high signal intensity throughout the colon whereas all surrounding tissues remain low in signal intensity.

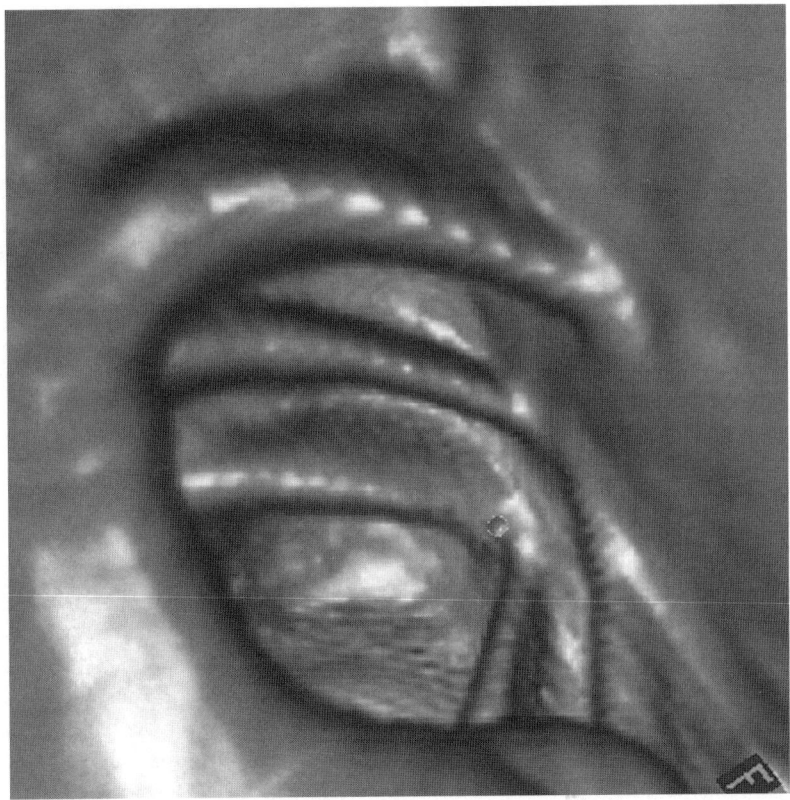

FIGURE 7.4. A high contrast between the contrast-filled colonic lumen and surrounding structures is the basis for subsequent virtual colonic viewing.

A complete analysis of an MRC exam still requires 15 minutes of interactive image viewing on a high-performance workstation. In a first-step MRC, images should be interpreted in the multiplanar reformation mode scrolling through the prone 3D dataset in all three orthogonal planes. In regions containing larger pockets of residual air, the assessment needs to be supplemented by views of the supine dataset. In a second step, the data should be assessed based on virtual endoscopic renderings displaying the inside of the colonic lumen. A virtual endoscopic fly-through allows the observer to concentrate on the colon, facilitating depiction of small structures protruding into the colonic lumen. Further, the 3D depth perception allows the assessment of haustral fold morphology, thereby enhancing the observer's ability to distinguish polyps from haustra. To assure complete visualization of both sides of haustral folds, the virtual fly-through should be performed in an antegrade as well as retrograde direction.

Dark-Lumen MRC

The detection of colorectal lesions with bright-lumen MRC relies on the visualization of filling defects. Apart from polyps, differential considerations for such filling defects include air bubbles and residual fecal material. To differentiate these possibilities, datasets are collected in both the prone and supine patient positions: Air and fecal material move, while polyps remain stationary. While effective in most instances, the technique can introduce errors. Thus, polyps with a long stalk may move sufficiently to simulate a moving air bubble or residual stool, whereas stool adherent to the colonic wall may not move at all, thereby simulating a polyp. In addition to obviating the need for a second, time-consuming 3D data acquisition set, dark-lumen MRC facilitates the identification of polyps.

Dark-lumen MRC is based on contrast generated between a brightly enhancing colonic wall and a homogeneously dark colonic lumen (Lauenstein et al. 2001). The technique differs from bright-lumen MRC in the following manner:

1. Instead of a gadolinium containing enema, only tap water is administered rectally, rendering low signal on heavily T1-weighted 3D GRE acquisitions.
2. The colonic filling process is monitored with a fluoroscopic T2W sequence rather than a T1W sequence.
3. To obtain a bright colonic wall, paramagnetic contrast is administered intravenously. 3D data sets are collected prior to giving the paramagnetic contrast agent and after a 75-second delay.
4. Because residual air exhibits no signal in the colonic lumen, the examination needs to be performed only in the prone patient position.

Compared to bright-lumen MRC, which has been extensively evaluated in the past, dark-lumen MRC harbors considerable advantages, including reduced examination and postprocessing times, because only one 3D dataset needs to be collected. Further, the dark-lumen technique copes with the problem of residual stool in a simple manner: If the lesion enhances, it is a polyp; if it does not enhance, it represents stool (Figs 7.5 and 7.6). Suspicious-appearing lesions are an-

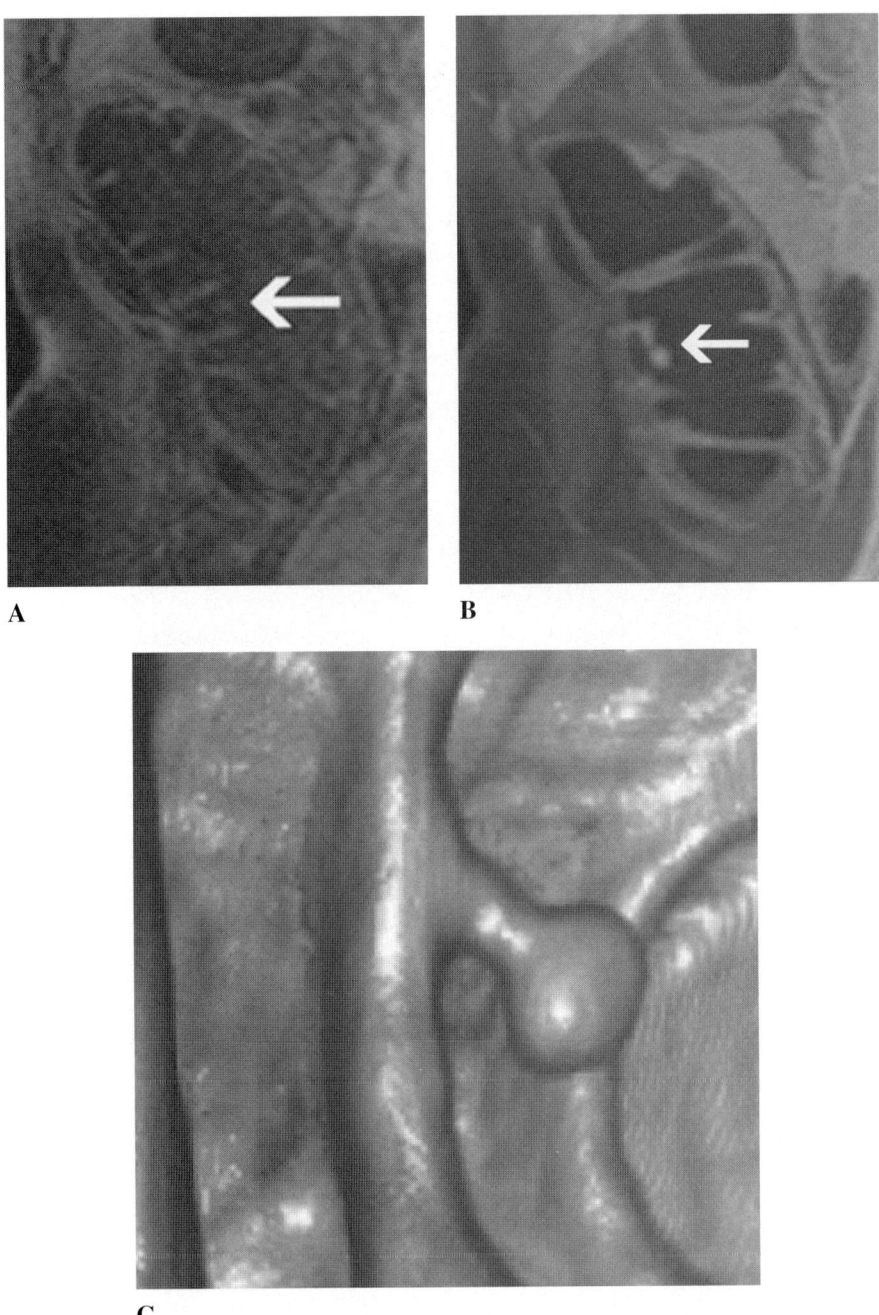

A   B

C

FIGURE 7.5. A 10-mm polyp could be detected in the ascending colon based on the contrast uptake (arrow, **B**) compared to the corresponding native sequence (arrow, **A**). Diagnosis was confirmed by virtual endoscopic rendering (**C**) as well as conventional colonoscopy.

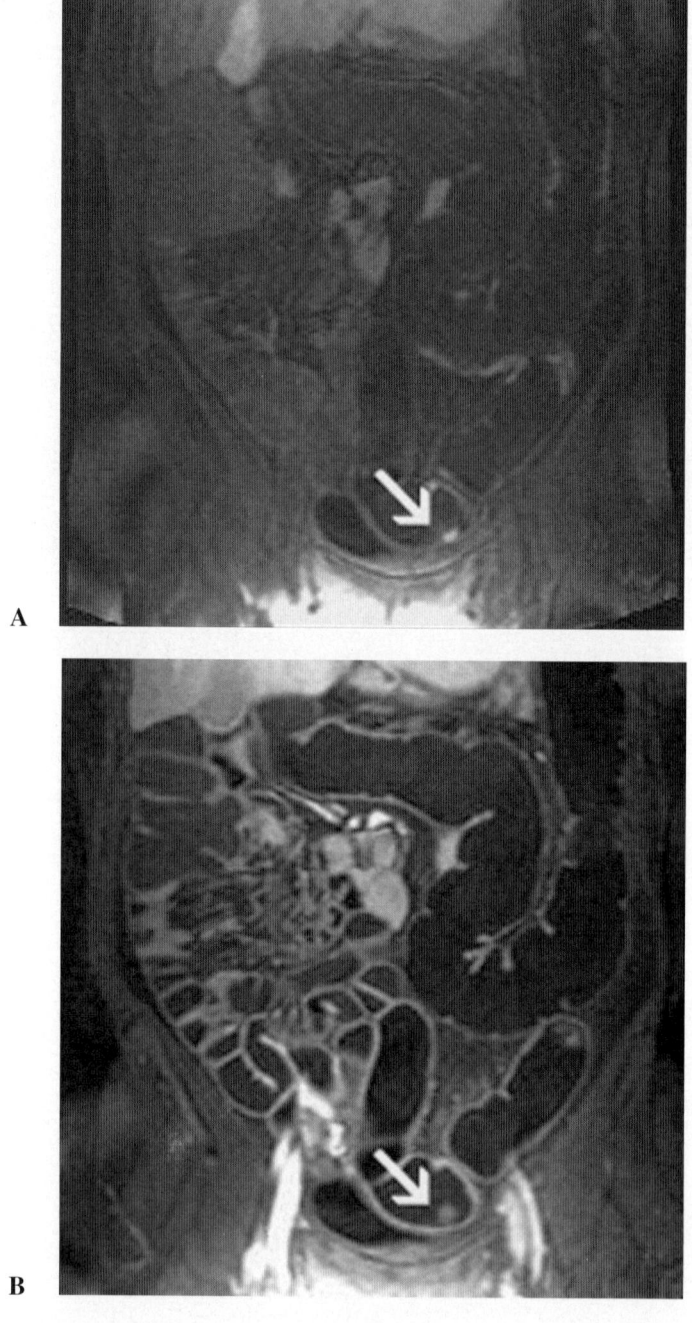

FIGURE 7.6. Polyp-simulating protrusion in the sigmoid colon (arrow, **B**) turned out to be residual stool because of the same signal intensity compared to native scan (arrow, **A**). Subsequent conventional colonoscopy confirmed absence of colorectal pathologies.

alyzed by comparing signal intensities on the pre- and postcontrast images. If the analysis were limited to the postcontrast dataset, bright stool could be misinterpreted as a polyp. Comparison with the precontrast images documents the lack of contrast enhancement, securing the correct diagnosis.

Enhancement of colorectal masses following the IV administration of contrast material has been documented in conjunction with MRC (Luboldt et al. 1998) and CTC (Morrin et al. 2000). The use of intravenously administered contrast material significantly improves reader confidence in the assessment of bowel wall conspicuity and the ability to depict medium-sized polyps in suboptimally prepared colons. The enhancement observed within polyps exceeds enhancement of the colonic wall. This may aid in differentiating even very small polyps from thickened haustral folds.

A further advantage of dark-lumen MRC relates to the fact that it permits direct analysis of the bowel wall. This facilitates the evaluation of inflammatory changes in patients with inflammatory bowel disease (Fig 7.7). Increased contrast uptake and bowel wall thickening, as documented on contrast-enhanced T_1-weighted images, has already been shown to correlate well with the degree of inflammation in the small bowel (Marcos and Semelka 2000). Hence, the dark-

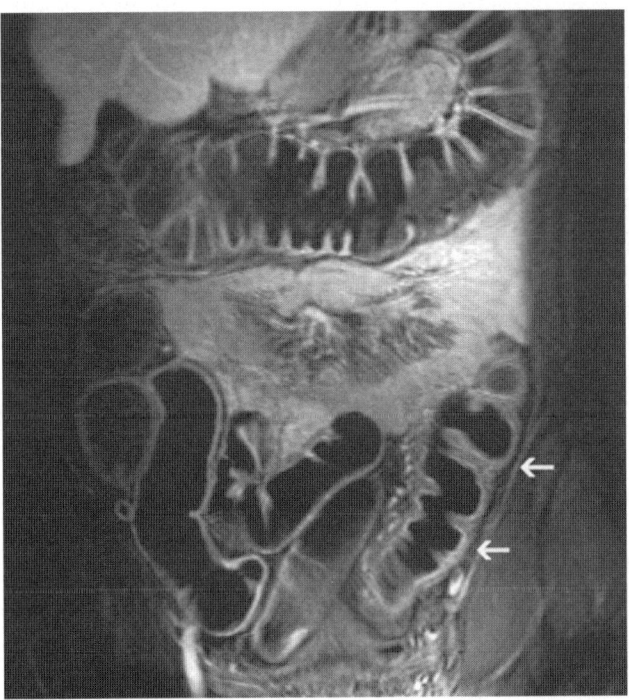

FIGURE 7.7. Increased contrast enhancement and thickened bowel wall in the descending colon (arrows) as a sign for an inflammatory lesion in a patient with Crohn's disease.

lumen approach may indeed amplify the list of indications for MRC in the future to also encompass inflammatory bowel disease.

Finally, the IV application of paramagnetic contrast agents permits a more comprehensive assessment of parenchymal abdominal organs contained within the field of view. By combining pre- and postcontrast T_1-weighted imaging, the liver can be accurately evaluated regarding the presence and type of concomitant pathology. Dark-lumen MRC also offers new perspectives regarding optimization of bowel distention. Although the administration of water as a rectal enema does not adversely affect patient comfort in most cases, a modified strategy could be based on the application of gases like CO_2 (Lomas et al. 2001) or room air (Morrin et al. 2001). Gas has no signal and would thus easily permit delineation of the contrast-enhanced colonic wall and masses. This approach has been shown to be feasible in smaller patient groups (Lomas et al. 2001; Morrin et al. 2001).

Diagnostic Accuracy

The diagnostic performance of bright-lumen MRC was assessed in several studies (Luboldt et al. 2000; Saar et al. 2000) using conventional colonoscopy as the standard of reference. While most mass lesions smaller than 5 mm were missed (Luboldt et al. 2000), almost all lesions exceeding 10 mm were correctly identified (Table 7.1). In a study by Pappalardo et al. (2000), MRC even detected a higher total number of polyps exceeding 10 mm than conventional colonoscopy. MRC identified additional polyps in regions of the colon not reached by colonoscopy.

Direct observational data on growth rates indicated that polyps smaller than 10 mm remain stable over 3 years and are not prone to malignant degradation (Villavicencio and Rex 2000). Hence, bright-lumen MRC may be considered al-

TABLE 7.1. Accuracy of MRC compared to conventional colonoscopy.

All lesions	
Sensitivity	27/58 = 47%
Specificity	48/59 = 81%
PPV	27/38 = 71%
NPV	48/79 = 61%
Lesions >10 mm	
Sensitivity	13/14 = 93%
Specificity	102/103 = 99%
PPV	13/14 = 93%
NPV	102/103 = 99%

Source: Adapted with permission from Luboldt et al. (2000). PPV, positive-predictive valve; NPV, negative-predictive valve.

most as reliable as conventional colonoscopy for the assessment of colonic lesions at risk for malignant degeneration. Nevertheless, attempts are underway to increase the spatial resolution of the underlying 3D datasets and thereby improve the diagnostic accuracy of MRC for lesions ranging from 5 to 10 mm. Technical refinements include the use of even shorter repetition times in conjunction with zero filling routines and the implementation of parallel imaging routines (Griswold et al. 2000).

Fecal Tagging

MRC still requires bowel cleansing in a manner similar to conventional colonoscopy. Because 75% of patients undergoing bowel preparation complain about symptoms ranging from feeling unwell to inability to sleep (Elwood et al. 1995), patient acceptance is negatively impacted. To assure high patient acceptance of MRC, bowel cleansing needs to be eliminated. This can be accomplished with fecal tagging—a concept based on modulating the signal intensity of fecal material by adding contrast compounds to regular meals.

Fitting the two approaches to MRC (bright lumen and dark lumen), there are also two theoretical approaches to fecal tagging. Its principle was demonstrated on the basis of a bright rectal enema distending the colonic lumen containing brightly tagged stool in conjunction with bright-lumen MRC (Weishaupt et al. 1999). By adding a T_1-shortening Gd-based MR contrast agent to regular meals prior to the MR examination, harmonization of signal properties between fecal material and the Gd-based enema was achieved. The oral administration of a paramagnetic MR contrast agent (Gd-DOTA) has been shown to be safe. The combination of fecal tagging with a paramagnetic contrast agent and colonic filling results in a homogeneous signal distribution throughout the colon (Fig 7.8). In these examinations, virtual MRC allows an unobstructed view through the colon because the tagged stool is virtually indistinguishable from the administered enema. Although encouraging results concerning acceptance and image interpretation were obtained, the clinical implementation of bright-lumen fecal tagging was hindered by the high cost of the Gd-based paramagnetic contrast agent.

A second strategy for fecal tagging is based on rendering the colonic lumen dark (Lauenstein et al. 2001). For fecal tagging, a highly concentrated barium sulfate containing contrast agent (Micropaque; Guerbet, Sulzbach, Germany; 1g barium sulfate/mL) is administered in a volume of 200 mL with each of four principle meals beginning 36 hours prior to MRC. Patients are instructed to avoid the intake of all fiber-rich foodstuff and nourishments with high concentration of manganese, such as chocolate or fruits, during this period, because manganese leads to increased signal intensity on T1w sequences. "Barium-based" fecal tagging is combined with dark-lumen MRC: The colon is distended with a rectally administered water enema and a paramagnetic contrast agent is

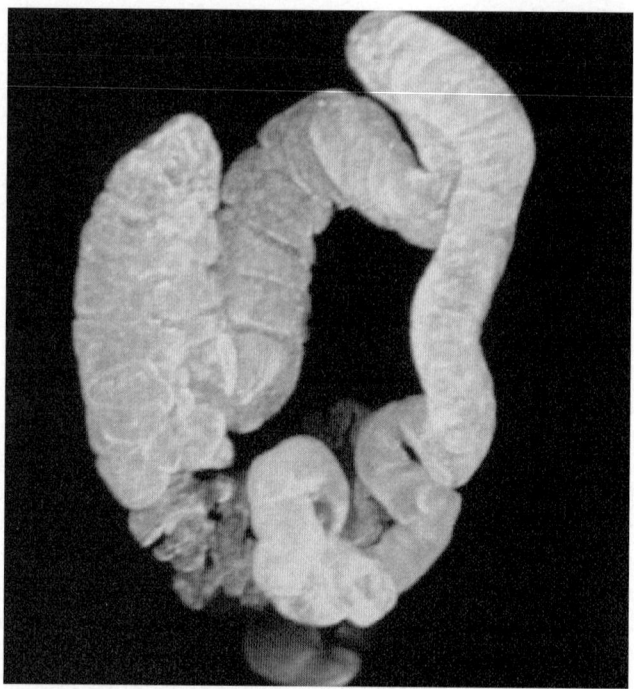

FIGURE 7.8. MIP display of a 3D MRC dataset collected following gadolinium-based fecal tagging (left). After filling the colon with a gadolinium-containing enema, the tagged stool is no longer seen because its signal intensity is similar to that of the applied rectal gadolinium/water enema.

administered intravenously to render the colonic wall and adherent colorectal mass lesions bright.

Barium sulfate is a well-known diagnostic contrast agent, still in common use as an oral agent for esophageal, gastric, and small-bowel radiography. Compared to Gd-based contrast compounds, it is far less costly and characterized by an even better safety profile. Anaphylactoid reactions or other adverse side effects are virtually unknown. The agent is not absorbed and mixes well with stool. Thus, barium includes all characteristics as an ideal oral tagging agent for MRC.

The barium-based approach to fecal tagging has been successfully employed. The signal-reducing effects upon stool have been documented in volunteer studies. By ingesting barium prior to the MR examination, stool is rendered virtually indistinguishable from the administered water enema on heavily T1w 3D GRE images (Figs 7.7 and 7.9). The MR examination without prior ingestion of barium reveals signal-rich stool, which cannot readily be differentiated from the brightly enhancing colonic wall (Fig 7.10).

Recently, the barium-based fecal tagging concept has been successfully evaluated in a pilot patient study. Fecal tagged MRC revealed all polyps larger than

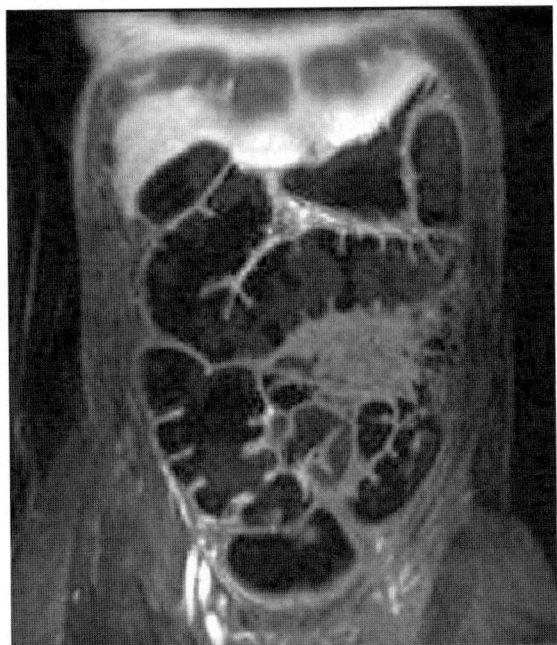

FIGURE 7.9. MRC in conjunction with barium sulfate-based fecal tagging. The colonic wall is bright because of the IV application of Gd-DTPA, whereas the barium-containing enema and the barium-tagged stool render the colonic lumen dark.

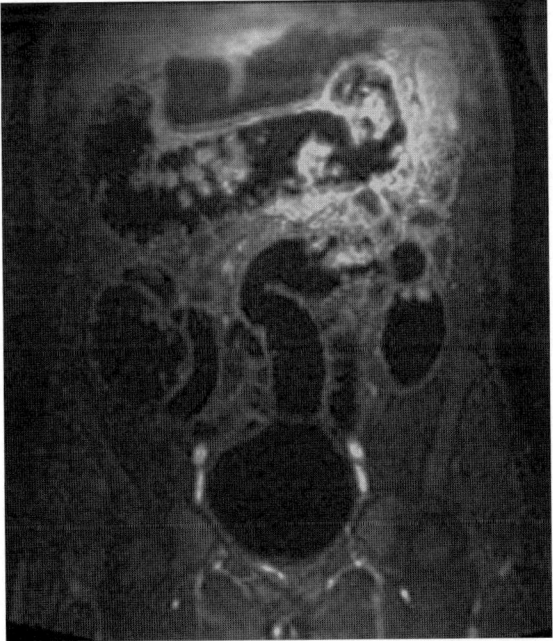

FIGURE 7.10. Dark-lumen MRC without fecal tagging and without prior bowel cleansing. Signal-rich stool in the transverse colon cannot be differentiated from the brightly enhancing colonic wall, so a reliable exclusion of colonic pathologies is not possible.

8 mm in a population of 24 patients with known or suspected colorectal tumors (Lauenstein et al. 2002). The overall sensitivity of MRC was 89.3% for the detection of colorectal masses and the specificity was 100%. Although further work is required to confirm these results, it seems that barium-tagged MRC may well emerge as the examination strategy of choice for the early detection of polyps in asymptomatic subjects. The technique appears to combine excellent diagnostic accuracy with high patient acceptance based on a painless examination and no need for colonic cleansing.

8

Future Directions:
Computer-Aided Diagnosis

Ronald M. Summers and Hiroyuki Yoshida

While significant progress is being made with clinical evaluation of computed tomography (CT) colonography (CTC), the issues of cost, time for interpretation, diagnostic performance, and perceptual error have yet to be addressed. A number of researchers around the world have embarked on a project to develop computer-aided diagnosis (CAD) of colonic polyps to address these potential obstacles to further use of CTC. In this chapter, we briefly review the progress to date and speculate on developments likely to occur during the next few years.

Progress to Date

CAD is a diagnosis made by radiologists who take into account computer output as an aid, guide, or second opinion. The final diagnosis is made by radiologists. Although, in general, CAD is not restricted to a detection task (i.e., CAD can potentially characterize lesions), to date most CAD schemes for CTC are limited to automated detection only.

Building upon their prior work in virtual bronchoscopy, Summers et al. (1998, 2000b) presented work on computer-aided detection of colonic polyps with a CTC dataset augmented with simulated polyps. These simulated polyps were shown in a separate study to mimic the size, shape, and location of actual polyps with CTC (Beaulieu et al. 1998). In their shape-based algorithm, the computer calculates the local shape of each small portion of the surface of the colon and looks for areas that protrude inward toward the lumen like a polyp (Fig 8.1; see color insert) (Summers et al. 2000b, 2001). This computer technique ignores portions of the colonic wall shaped like haustral folds or normal colonic mucosa. More than 95% of the colonic wall could be eliminated from further analysis using this first-pass algorithm. Further refinement of the algorithm requires the use of thresholds on quantitative indices of shape, such as "Gaussian curvature" and a quantitative determination of the "sphericity" or sphere-like nature of the potential polyp. With these additional criteria, more than 99% of the colonic surface can be eliminated from further analysis. Of 10 simulated polyps placed in

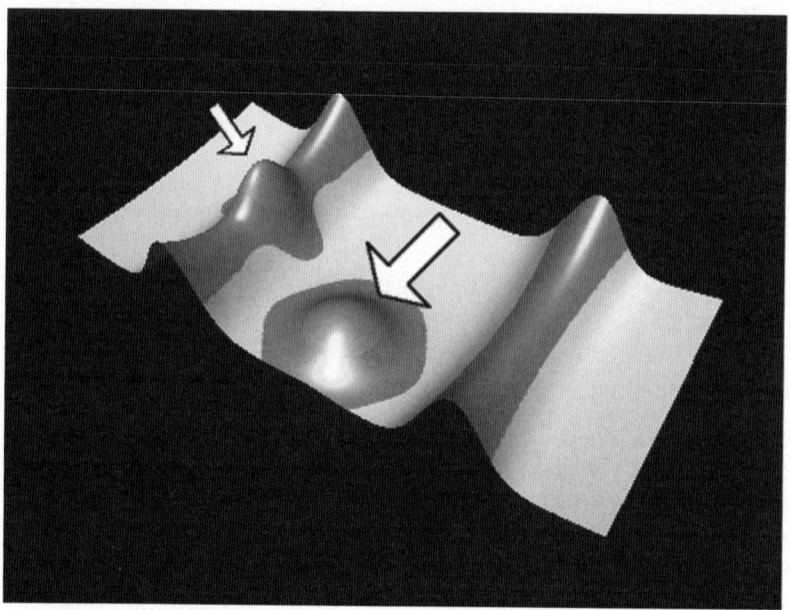

FIGURE 8.1. Conceptual diagram of colonic surface shape showing haustral folds (green), polyps (orange-red), and normal colonic surface between folds (yellow). A polyp on a fold (small arrow) and one between folds (large arrow) are shown. Polyps can be distinguished from folds and normal colonic mucosa by their distinctive shapes. (Used with permission from Summers 2000b.) (See color insert)

the CTC dataset, 8 could be detected with no false positive diagnoses (Summers et al. 2000b).

Summers further applied these earlier results to 20 CTC datasets having at least one polyp 1 cm or larger per patient (Summers et al. 2001c). They showed that 64% (18/28) polyps 1 cm or larger could be detected (Fig 8.2; see color insert). Moreover, when only polyps in well-distended colonic segments were considered the fraction of detected polyps increased to 71%. The average number of false positive detections was approximately six per patient. When the CT attenuation of the possible polyp was considered, the number of false positives dropped to an average of 3.5. Their software marked potential polyps directly on the CTC images to ease clinical interpretation (Summers et al. 2000).

Yoshida et al. (Yoshida and Nappi 2001, Yoshida et al. 2002a, b) developed a CAD scheme based on 3D volumetric feature analysis, which also relied to a great extent on analysis of shape. This scheme consists of three major steps: extraction of the colon, detection of polyp candidates, and elimination of false positive detections. In the first step, a thick region containing the entire colonic wall is extracted from an isotropic volumetric dataset generated from CTC images (Nappi and Yoshida 2002; Masutani et al. 2001) (Fig 8.3). Polyp candidates are detected from the thick region by extraction of a geometric feature called the vol-

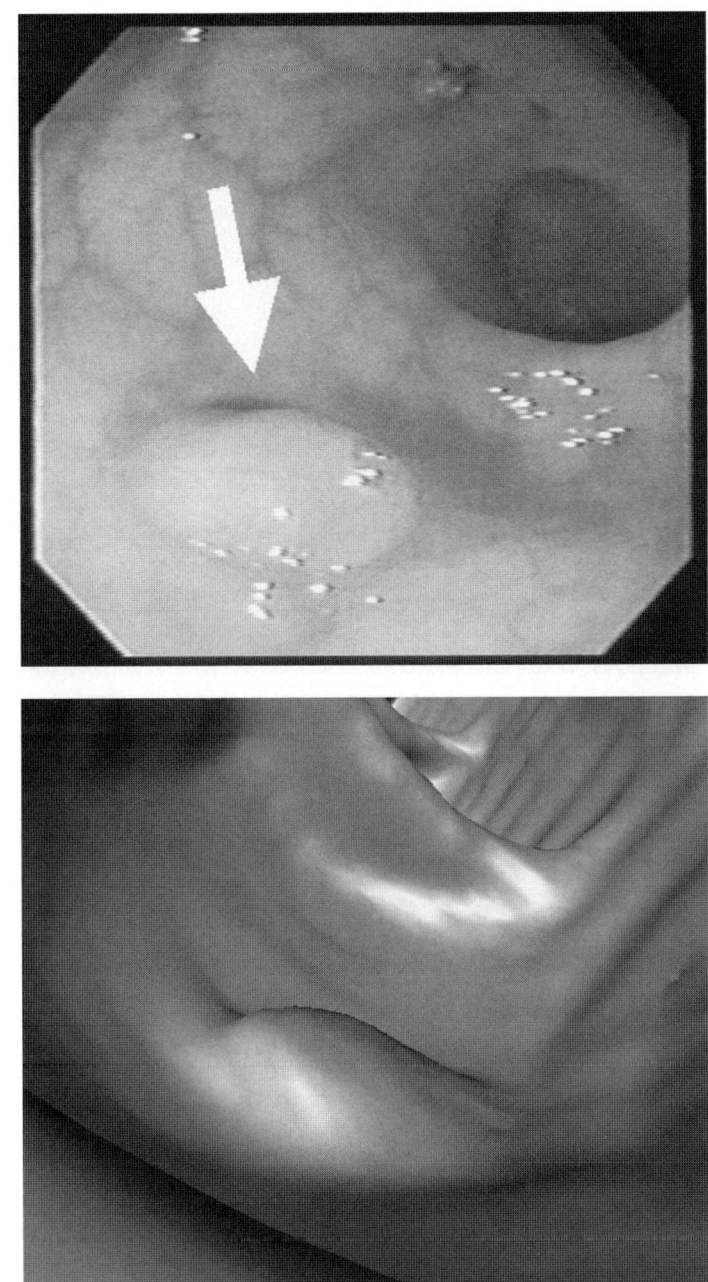

A

B

FIGURE 8.2. Examples of three polyps (arrows) measuring 1 to 1.5 cm. (**A, C, E**) Conventional colonoscopy and (**B, D, F**) corresponding CTC perspective renderings. (**B, D, F**), Red indicates portion of polyps detected by computer-assisted detection algorithm. Note the absence of false positive diagnoses on folds and normal colonic mucosa. (Used with permission from Summers et al. 2001c.) (See color insert)

Continues on next page

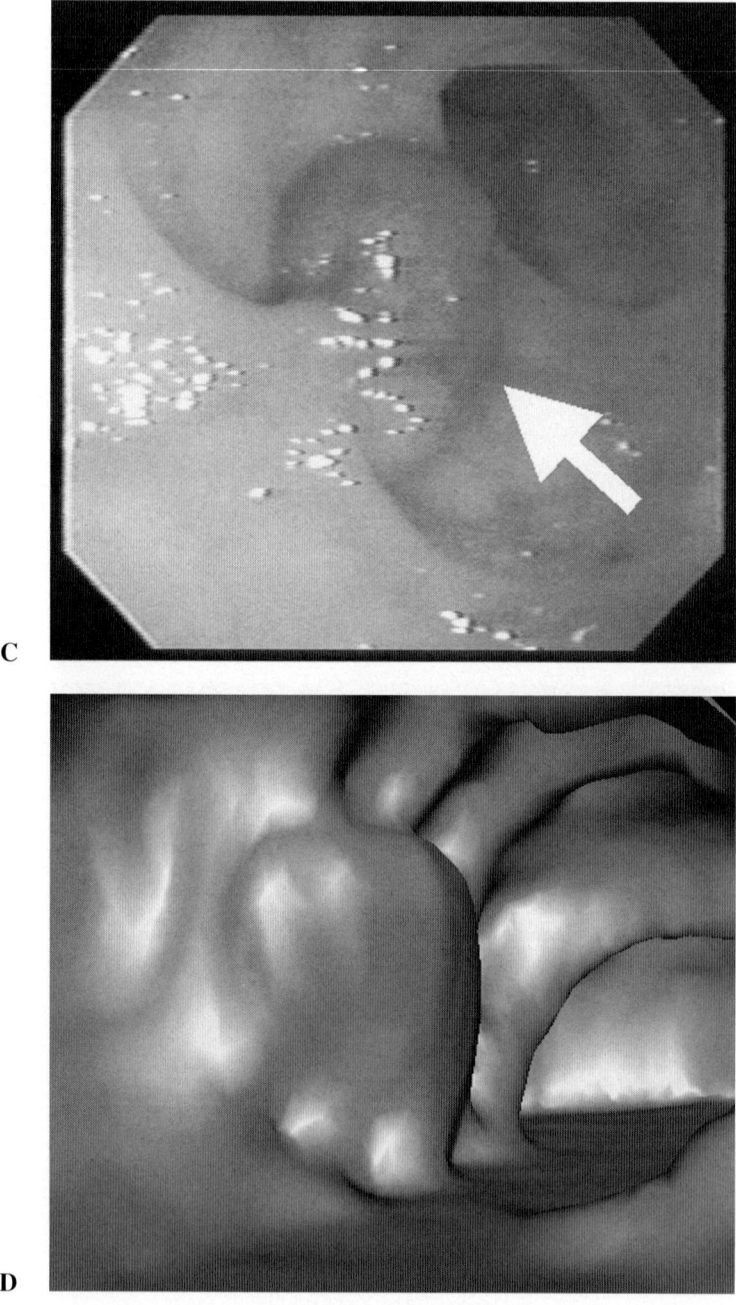

C

D

FIGURE 8.2. (*Continued*)

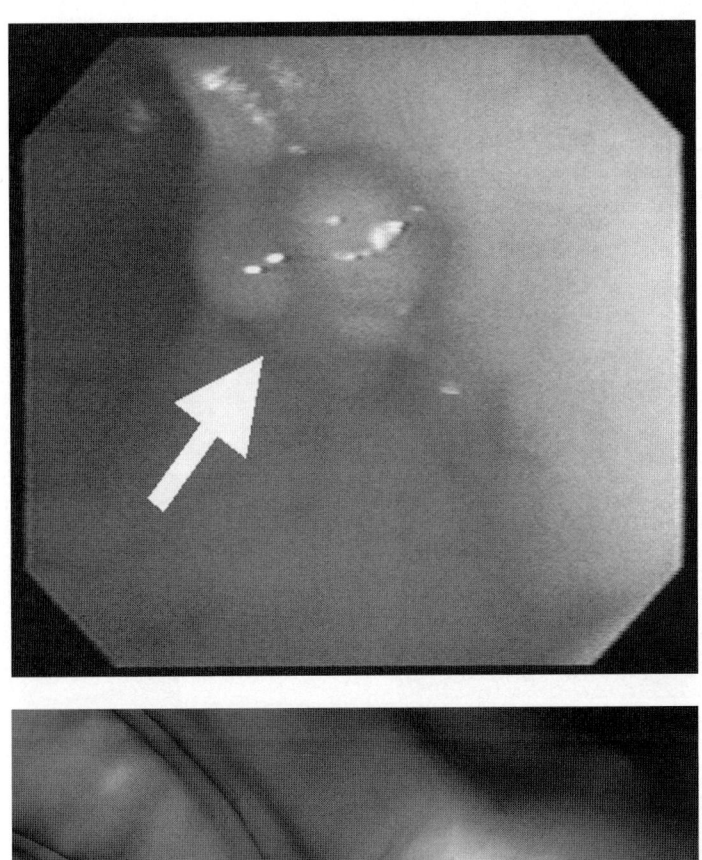

E

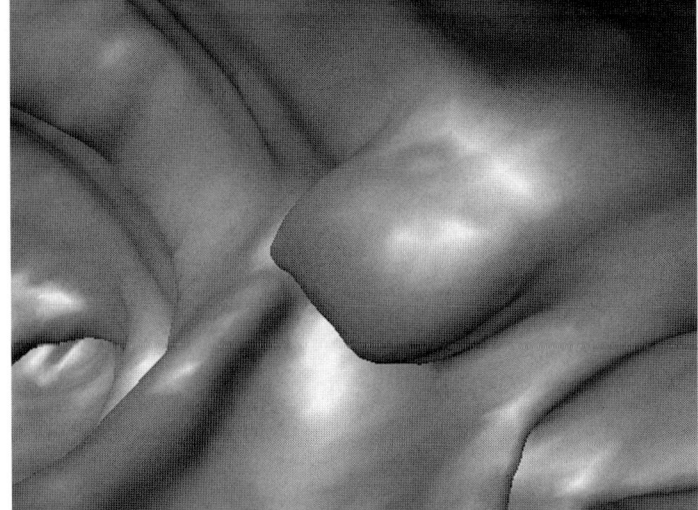

F

FIGURE 8.2. (*Continued*)

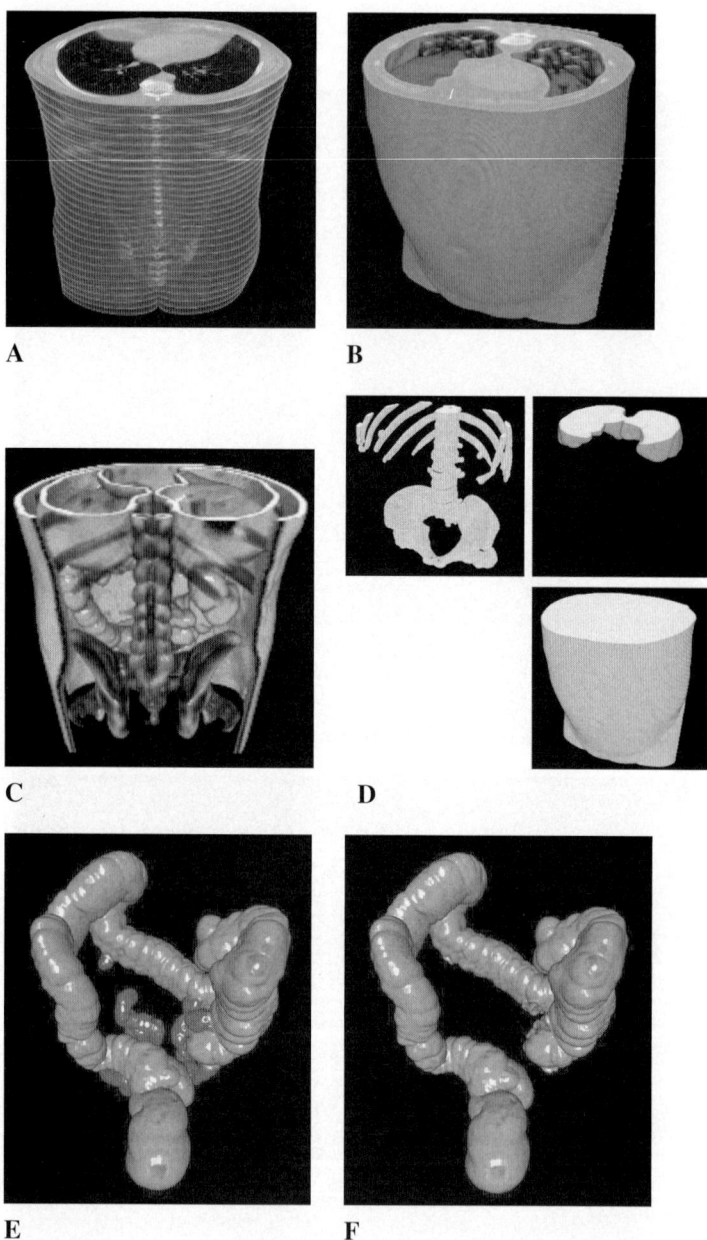

FIGURE 8.3. Extraction of the colon based on a knowledge-guided approach. (**A**) Original axial CT slices obtained from a CTC examination. (**B**) Isotropic volumetric data set generated by interpolation between the CT images in (**A**) along the longitudinal direction. (**C**) Anatomic structures obtained by application of thresholding operation to CT values in the volumetric data set in (**B**). (**D**) Example of extracolonic structures extracted from (**C**). In clockwise order from the upper-left corner: the osseous structures (spine, pelvis, parts of the ribs), the lung bases, and the body. (**E**) Colon extracted from (**C**) by removal of the extracolonic structures in (**D**). Parts of the small bowel (red) adhering to the colon are extracted along with the colon. (**F**) Final extracted colon (a thick region containing the entire colonic wall) after the removal of the small bowel. (Used with permission from Yoshida and Nappi 2001.)

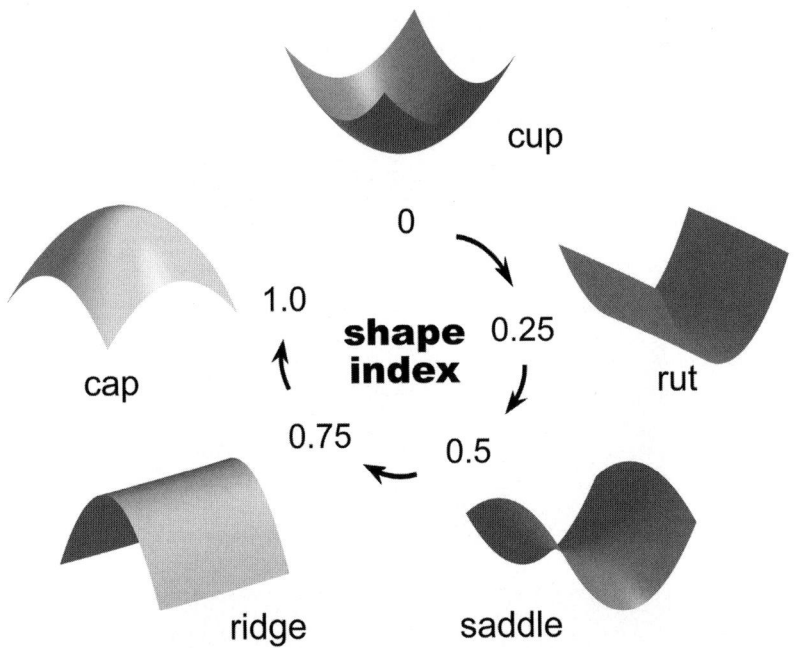

FIGURE 8.4. Relationship between the volumetric shape index values and shape classes. Polyps tend to appear as bulbous, cap-like structures adhering to the colonic wall, and thus have a shape index value close to 1. Folds appear as elongated, ridge-like structures, and have a shape index value of approximately 0.75. The colonic wall appears as a large, nearly flat, cup-like structure, and has a shape index value of close to 0. By coloring voxels that have shape index values corresponding to the cap, saddle to ridge, and the other classes by green, pink, and brown, respectively, one can distinguish these structures clearly (see Fig 8.5). (Used with permission from Yoshida, Masutani, and MacEneaney et al. 2002.) (See color insert)

umetric shape index at each voxel. Every distinct shape corresponds to a unique value of the shape index (Fig 8.4; see color insert). In general, polyps tend to appear as bulbous, cap-like structures adhering to the colonic wall; folds appear as elongated, ridge-like structures; and the colonic wall appears as a nearly flat, cup-like structure. Therefore, the shape index can differentiate among polyps, folds, and the colonic wall (Fig 8.5; see color insert). False positives are distinguished from true positives by means of their geometric and textural features. The CAD scheme was evaluated in 71 CTC cases, including 14 cases having 21 colonoscopy-confirmed polyps >5 mm (Yoshida et al. 2002). There were 15 polyps ≤10 mm and 6 polyps >10 mm. In a by-patient analysis, the sensitivity was 100% with an average false positive rate of 2.0 per patient; in other words, the scheme found at least 1 polyp in all of the 15 polyp cases. In a by-polyp analysis, the CAD scheme detected 90% (19/21) of the polyps at the same false positive rate. The types of false positives were similar to those due to common per-

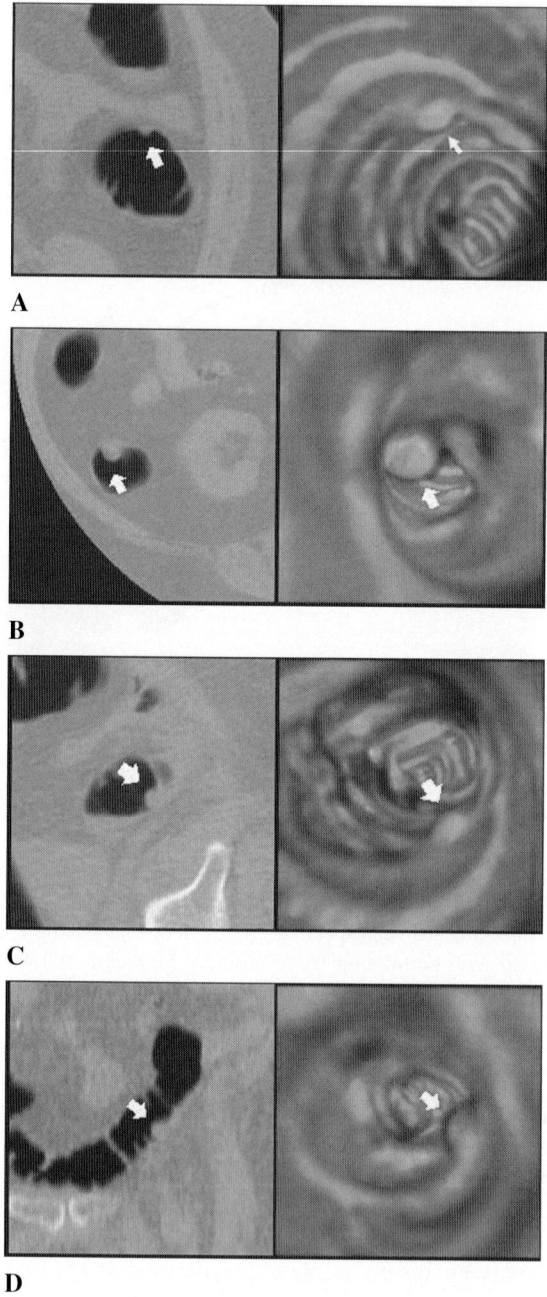

FIGURE 8.5. Effect of the volumetric shape index in differentiation among polyps, folds, and the colonic wall. In each pair of images, an axial or coronal CT image that contains a polyp indicated by arrow is shown on the left and its 3D endoscopic views by perspective volume rendering is shown on the right: (**A**) 6-mm polyp in sigmoid, (**B**) 9-mm polyp in sigmoid, (**C**) 8-mm polyp in sigmoid, (**D**) 9-mm polyp in sigmoid. With the coloring scheme shown in Fig 8.4, polyps, folds, and the colonic wall are clearly separated, and the polyps are easily distinguishable from other structures. (Used with permission from Yoshida, Nappi, and MacEneaney et al. 2002; Yoshida and Nappi 2001.) (See color insert)

ceptual errors for radiologists. However, most of these false positives were easily distinguishable from polyps by experienced radiologists.

Paik et al. (1999) used a Canny edge detector and the Hough transform (HT) as their first-pass polyp detector (Paik et al. 1999). The HT locates possible polyps by identifying spherical surfaces on the colon. Available data are limited to abstracts, but they reported sensitivities as high as 92.9% and 7.9 false positives per colon for a dataset encompassing 14 polyps >8.5 mm in 9 patients (Paik et al. 2001). In a recent refinement, Göktürk et al. (2001) proposed the use of the random orthogonal shape section (ROSS) method, a statistical pattern recognition approach that reduces the false positive rate by 62%. The ROSS method examines a large number of subvolumes in the vicinity of a possible polyp, generates shape signatures based on lines, circles, and quadratics fit to the inner colonic wall edge, and then feeds the signatures into "support vector machines," a form of classifier (Göktürk et al. 2001).

Vining et al. (1999) also reported a computer-assisted polyp detection algorithm. Their algorithm combined surface curvature and wall thickness assessment, identified and rejected haustral folds, and then ranked detections based on the product of a group convexity value, height measurement, and number of vertices comprising a lesion. Their CAD software identified 11 of 15 polyps in 10 patients.

These early results show that CAD is capable of detecting polyps in CTC with reasonable false negative and false positive rates.

Future Work

As can be seen from the preceding section, CAD for CTC is an evolving field. Additional improvements in CAD can be expected in a number of areas although there are many challenges that must be overcome (Summers 2002). The most promising avenues of research, discussed in the section that follows, are in the following areas: bowel preparation, technical improvements in CAD, image resolution, clinical evaluation, and databases. Relevance of CAD to cancer detection and cost issues are also briefly described in this section.

Effect of Bowel Preparation

Considerable excitement has recently been generated by the application of stool subtraction techniques (Zalis and Hahn 2001; Chen et al. 2000). For subtraction, a patient is given an oral contrast agent such as a barium pill or solution or a water-soluble contrast agent. This is done 12 to 48 hours prior to the CTC procedure so that the contrast agent can mix with residual stool. Some researchers also give the patient a standard bowel preparation to cleanse the colon of the majority of the stool so that the tagging agent will opacify residual stool and fluid (Vining et al. 1999). Other researchers are investigating the "prepless" colon in which no cleansing of the bowel is necessary but the stool is tagged using an oral agent (Callstrom et al. 2001). In either case, stool tagging requires additional image processing techniques to eliminate the stool so that the physician can identify a polyp. Once the stool is subtracted, artifacts may be present due to the incompleteness of the stool subtraction algorithms. This will pose additional challenges for CAD and is a subject for future research.

Technical Improvements in CAD

While early results are promising, further improvements in CAD technology can be expected to increase the sensitivity and specificity of CTC. Three major areas for technical improvement are identification of image features that more directly distinguish true positives from false positives, improved classifiers to sort out the various features, and larger unbiased databases of CTC studies. That there is room for improvement is suggested by the fact that trained radiologists can identify 75% to 90% of polyps 1 cm or larger (Fenlon et al. 1999b; Yee et al. 2001; Fletcher et al. 2000); therefore, one might expect that it should be possible to teach a computer algorithm to have a similar performance. Currently, there appears to be a 20% to 30% gap between the performance of CAD and that of trained clinicians.

Effect of CT Scanning Parameters

Further research also needs to be done to determine the effects of different scanning parameters on the performance of CAD. For example, it is unknown at this time whether higher-resolution scans (greater longitudinal resolution) will improve the sensitivity and specificity of CTC. Because higher-resolution scans may come at the cost of increased image noise, determination of the effect of noise needs to be evaluated to determine how noise-tolerant CAD schemes can be.

Evaluation of CAD in the Clinical Setting

The integration of CAD into clinical practice will pose additional challenges. It will be important to show that the improved performance of CAD in the laboratory can be confirmed in a clinical setting. Observer performance studies (Metz 1999) should be conducted for evaluation of the diagnostic performance of a radiologist with and without computer aid in a prospective fashion to demonstrate the added benefit of CAD. Such studies have been conducted for CAD for mammography (Chan et al. 1999) and chest radiography (Kobayashi et al. 1996).

CAD and Cancer

At this time, it is thought that CAD will not be necessary for carcinoma detection. This assertion is supported by evidence from a series of seven published studies that reported that carcinomas were detected with 100% sensitivity (Summers et al. 2001). Cancers are often well visualized by the radiologist due to their size and invasiveness. In addition, cancers often have shape features much different from those of polyps, e.g., they may be circumferential or napkin-ring lesions. It may not be worth the effort to train the computer to detect such lesions. Consequently, research in the next few years is likely to focus primarily on polyp detection.

Processing Time

The speed of the computer algorithms may be an issue. As CTC data sets become larger as higher resolutions are used, the processing time will lengthen proportionally. For CAD to be a useful diagnostic aid, the most important time factor is the actual interpretation time by radiologists when they are aided by the computer output. To reduce interpretation time and improve the diagnostic performance of radiologists, CAD algorithms may therefore run in the background and their final output, such as locations of suspicious polyps and the likelihood of being a polyp, should be presented in real time.

Cost of CAD

The cost of CAD may be of concern if it is not reimbursed. In mammography, recent legislation has provided for a small fee for CAD. Until reimbursement is available, it is uncertain whether CAD will be commercialized even if it is shown to be robust in the laboratory and accurate in clinical research. Intellectual property issues may also arise as early researchers seek to gain the high ground and patent their algorithms for CAD.

Common Image Database

The American College of Radiology Imaging Network (ACRIN, www.acrin.org) is investigating the possibility of creating an image database for CAD for CTC. Such a database would consist of well-annotated cases, validated with the gold standards of conventional colonoscopy and pathology, and include demographic information about the subjects, such as age, gender, risk factors, and serum and stool markers. This resource could allow for a quantum leap in the speed at which CAD for CTC comes to fruition. Whereas CAD for mammography took 10 to 15 years to advance from concept to commercial product, CAD for CTC may come to market much faster because of the breadth of knowledge and the excellent foundation laid by researchers in other areas of CAD in radiology.

Conclusion

In summary, CAD for CTC has been shown to be feasible in early laboratory and clinical trials. Better clinical studies to show robustness are needed. There are a number of promising areas for future research that are likely to yield exciting results in the years to come.

9

A Word About Radiation Dose

James A. Brink

The development of computed tomography (CT) colonography (CTC) as a viable clinical tool has paralleled the rapid advancement of CT technology. About one decade after CT was revolutionized by the advent of spiral/helical CT technology, multislice CT (MDCT) was introduced, offering better longitudinal and temporal resolution. These benefits improve nearly all imaging applications in which broad anatomic coverage is required in a breath hold, including CTC. Although dual or split detector systems have been available since the early 1990s, CT scanners with four data channels were introduced in 1998 and have provided another quantum leap in CT performance, permitting thinner slices, shorter scans, and greater volume coverage. Now, systems with 8 to 16 data channels are emerging, and manufacturers are testing incorporation of flat-panel detectors in CT scanners as a future means of extending this technology to nearly instantaneous CT data acquisition. However, the potential for increased radiation exposure with MDCT has dampened enthusiasm for its use, in particular in screening applications such as CTC.

MDCT: Radiation Dose Considerations

The width of the radiation profile with MDCT is increased substantially relative to single-slice CT (SDCT), largely related to the use of cone beam rather than fan beam geometry. For MDCT scanners, the width of the radiation beam typically exceeds the total scan width, whereas for SDCT the radiation beam width is typically within 1 mm of the nominal scan width. This effect is amplified by the detector configuration used for any given scan. With the first release of a four-channel MDCT scanner (Lightspeed QX/i version 1.0, General Electric Co, Milwaukee), the radiation profile width exceeded the scan width by 150% (12.5 mm) for a nominal scan width of 5 mm (4 × 1.25-mm detector configuration). However, when the scan width was set to 20 mm (4- × 5-mm detector configuration), the radiation profile width exceeded the scan width by only 30% (26 mm) (McCullough and Zink 1999). As a result, for multislice body CT the maximum surface CTDI values increase by 76% for the 4- × 5-mm detector configuration and 238% for the 4- × 1.25-mm detector configuration, as compared to SDCT. Thus, when the full longitudinal extent of the detector is employed (4- × 5-mm detector configuration) the dose inefficiency of MDCT is minimized.

The difference in technique and radiation dose between SDCT and MDCT of the adult abdomen and pelvis has been well summarized by McCollough and Zink (1999). These investigators found that the scan time was reduced from 34 seconds to 16 seconds for 30 cm of coverage with a rotation time of 0.8 seconds by using MDCT (5-mm slice thickness, beam pitch of 0.75) as compared to SDCT (7-mm slice thickness, beam pitch of 1). Holding image noise constant, these authors also found that the tube current could be reduced from 310 mA to 190 mA by using MDCT for a total mAs of 10,540 for SDCT as compared to 3,040 for MDCT. However, despite this reduction in mAs, the radiation dose increase by approximately 50% at both the center and the surface of a 32-cm CTDI phantom, owing to the increased width of the radiation profile and a 25% overlap with MDCT (beam pitch of 0.75).

Subsequently, a focal spot tracking algorithm was developed to reduce such dose inefficiencies (Lightspeed QX/i, version 1.1). With this improvement, the maximum surface CTDI values for body MDCT increased by only 10% for the 4- × 5-mm detector configuration compared to 105% for the 4- × 1.25-mm detector configuration relative to CTDI values for SDCT. Although the maximum surface dose differential between MDCT and SDCT is minimized by use of the 4- × 5-mm detector configuration (10% difference), the effective dose (a measure related to the total energy deposited in the patient) was nearly equalized between MDCT and SDCT with this technique. This benefit is realized as a result of the elimination of overlap between scans performed during separate breath holds with SDCT by single breath hold examination with MDCT.

To further reduce dose with MDCT, one may consider replacing the 25% radiation overlap associated with a beam pitch of 0.75 with a 50% gap in the x-ray beam associated with a beam pitch of 1.5. However, most MDCT systems automatically adjust the tube current to maintain comparable levels of image noise, a feature that largely offsets any potential benefit to radiation dose associated with such an increase in pitch. A dose benefit may be realized only if one manually overrides this adjustment to reduce tube current, necessitating acceptance of an increased level of image noise (Mahesh et al. 2001). Although many imaging applications suffer degradation in diagnostic performance with increased levels of image noise, the diagnostic performance of high-contrast imaging applications such as CTC may not be degraded by such a change in technique. This is because the depiction of high-contrast interfaces between the air-filled lumen and the colon wall are not as subject to degradation by increased noise as are low-contrast imaging problems such as detection of subtle metastases within the liver.

The ability to image with thinner slices is one of the primary benefits of MDCT relative to SDCT. However, so long as image noise is held constant, radiation dose is necessarily increased to maintain photon flux as thinner sections are acquired. Although this applies to both SDCT and MDCT, a relative dose inefficiency is imparted with narrow-beam MDCT owing to the increased percentage of the x-ray beam that falls beyond the active detector rows (penumbra). Again, the tube current must be lowered, and an increased amount of image noise must be accepted when using thin-section MDCT. This practice is usually acceptable for high-contrast imaging applications such as CTC. In instances in which review of organs other than the colon is warranted, thicker sections may be generated by postprocessing thin slices into thicker reformations on an image review workstation or reconstructing thicker sections from a thin-slice acquisition, retrospectively. The increased noise associated with acquisition of thin-data slices at MDCT will be offset, in part, by either technique.

New innovations in radiation dose reduction continue to emerge that go beyond focal spot tracking techniques intended to minimize wasted radiation from the penumbra. Taking advantage of differences in patient thickness as the tube rotates around the patient, several manufacturers have sought to modulate the x-ray tube current synergistically with changes in patient thickness. Such an approach may result in substantial dose reduction benefits. As an extention of this technology, variations on patient thickness longitudinally may also be matched to alterations in x-ray beam intensity as the patient travels through the x-ray gantry. Together, these two beam modulation techniques synergistically reduce the radiation dose imparted to any given patient.

With the rapid acceptance of four-channel MDCT scanners, system designers have recently extended this technology to higher numbers of data channels that are active with each rotation of the gantry, increasing the number of data slices that may be acquired simultaneously. Four-channel MDCT units that were designed with a matrix detector configuration have had a small advantage in extending their standard design to permit acquisition of 8 and 16 data slices simultaneously. Because matrix detectors have detector elements that are all of equal size, detector row groupings may be easily reconfigured so as to permit acquisition of a larger number of slices with each rotation of the gantry. Conversely, four-channel MDCT systems that made use of an adaptive detector array in general required a redesign of the detector array to permit acquisition of a larger number of slices simultaneously, owing to the dissimilar size of the individual cells in the array. However, the radiation dose efficiency of matrix detectors tends to be less than the dose efficiency of adaptive detector arrays, owing to the attenuation of the x-ray beam by the numerous septae that divide the individual cells in the detector array.

One added advantage of increasing the number of data slices acquired simultaneously is an improvement in dose efficiency that results from a decrease in the amount of wasted radiation that falls beyond the active detector rows (penumbra). This is because greater longitudinal coverage is achieved with each rotation of the x-ray tube, permitting fewer instances in which the penumbra falls beyond the active detector rows. Siemens Medical Systems (Iselin, NJ) has reported an increase in dose utilization from 70% with 4- × 1-mm MDCT to more than 85% with 16- × 1.5-mm MDCT attributable to this geometric benefit.

CTC: Radiation Dose

Even before introduction of MDCT, radiation dose for CTC was a major concern. Investigators realized that trade-offs existed between resolution and radiation dose. Hara et al. (1997) first recognized that radiation dose with CTC may be reduced relative to conventional body CT examinations owing to the high-contrast imaging problem posed by detection of colonic polyps projecting into an air-filled lumen. These investigators showed that diagnostic performance was maintained despite a reduction in tube current from 140 mA to 70 mA with SDCT colonography, using 5-mm collimation and pitch of 1.3. The effective dose for combined supine and prone examinations was estimated to be 3.74 mGy for men and 5.70 mGy for women, approximately 50% lower than the radiation dose for a standard abdominal and pelvic CT scan, comparable to the radiation dose for a barium enema examination at their institution.

Moreover, investigators recognized that spatial resolution may be improved with thinner collumination and lower pitch settings with SDCT colonography. However, commensurate increases in radiation dose with high-resolution imaging posed a significant limitation. Springer et al. (2000) showed that the multiple-scan average dose increased from 6.9 mGy for SDCT colonography performed with 5-mm collimation and pitch of 2 to 15.2 mGy for SDCT colonography performed with 1-mm collimation and pitch of 1. However, such estimates were predicated on the assumption that increases in image noise would not be tolerable with use of thin-slice SDCT techniques. The transition to MDCT colonography prompted investigators to reconsider this notion.

Practically, two approaches have been advocated in design of protocols for CTC performed with MDCT. First, some investigators have sought to keep both image noise and radiation dose with MDCT colonography equivalent to that observed with SDCT colonography (Hara et al. 2001). By necessity, these investigators have chosen to use a slice thickness comparable to SDCT (5 mm) and a detector configuration that minimizes dose inefficiency (4 × 5 mm). When coupled with a beam pitch of 0.75 and a tube current of 50 mA, the effective dose is found to be nearly equivalent in MDCT and SDCT techniques (MDCT = 470 mrem and SDCT = 440 mrem in men; MDCT = 670 mrem and SDCT = 670 mrem in women). This protocol equivalency was determined with both in vivo and in vitro studies aimed at resolving 5-mm polyps while maintaining comparable levels of image noise for SDCT and MDCT (McCullough et al. 1999). However, such an approach does not take advantage of the inherent potential for improved resolution with MDCT as compared to SDCT.

Conversely, Macari, Bini, Milano et al. (2001) further explored the potential to improve spatial resolution with MDCT colonography while limiting radiation dose. By lowering the tube current and accepting a higher level of image noise, they performed high-resolution MDCT colonography with 4- × 1-mm detector configuration, a beam pitch of 1.5 to 1.75, and a gantry rotation period of 500 milliseconds. The tube current was limited to just 50 "effective" mAs. As such, they administered an effective dose of only 5 to 8 mSv for combined prone and supine examination as compared to 6 to 8 mSv for barium enema examinations. Scans were performed on the Siemens VolumeZoom MDCT scanner (Siemens Medical Systems). This scanner typically specifies the tube current in terms of effective mAs, which must be understood when translating this technique to other manufacturers. The effective mAs is calculated by multiplying the true tube current by the gantry rotation period and dividing by the beam pitch. Thus, the true tube current in this study was 150 mA for beam pitch of 1.5 and 500-millisecond gantry rotation period (50 effective mAs = 150 true mA × 0.5 s/1.5). Translating this technique to the GE MDCT scanner (Lightspeed QX/i, version 1.1), operating with 4- × 1.25-mm detector configuration, HS mode (beam pitch = 1.5), and 800-millisecond gantry rotation period, a true tube current of 100 mA corresponds to an effective mAs of 53 (53 effective mAs = 100 true mA × 0.8 s/1.5). As such, the effective dose for prone and supine examinations with this technique is 7.6 mSv. Although image noise is increased with this technique, Macari and colleagues showed that diagnostic performance was not degraded by such levels of image noise, and the advantage of high-resolution imaging was evident in improved definition of small polyps, in particular in regions of colonic tortuosity. Translation of this low-dose, high-resolution protocol to the GE Lightspeed CT scanner has proved similarly valuable as illustrated in Figure 9.1.

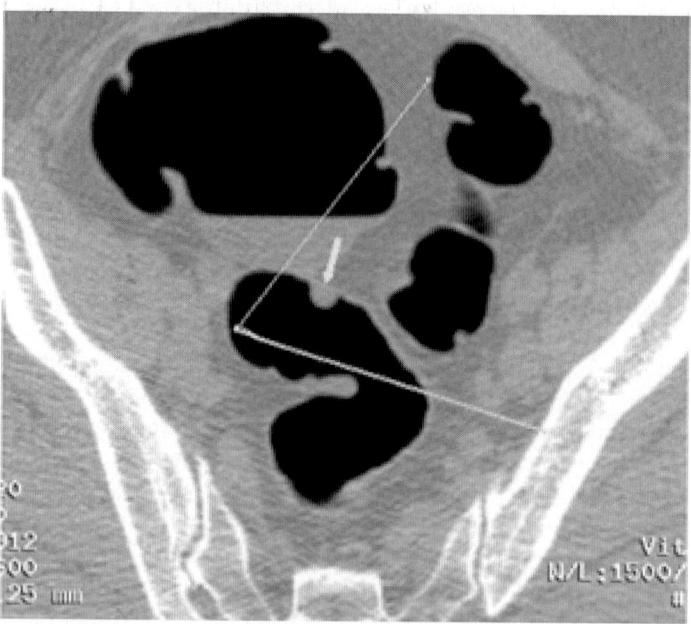

A

FIGURE 9.1. Low-dose, high-resolution CTC performed with 4- × 1.25-mm detector configuration, beam pitch of 1.5 at 120 kv and 100 mA using an 800-ms gantry rotation (Lightspeed QX/i, version 1.1). The effective mAs is 53 mAs with an estimated effective dose of 7.6 mSv for both prone and supine examination. (A) Transaxial source image.

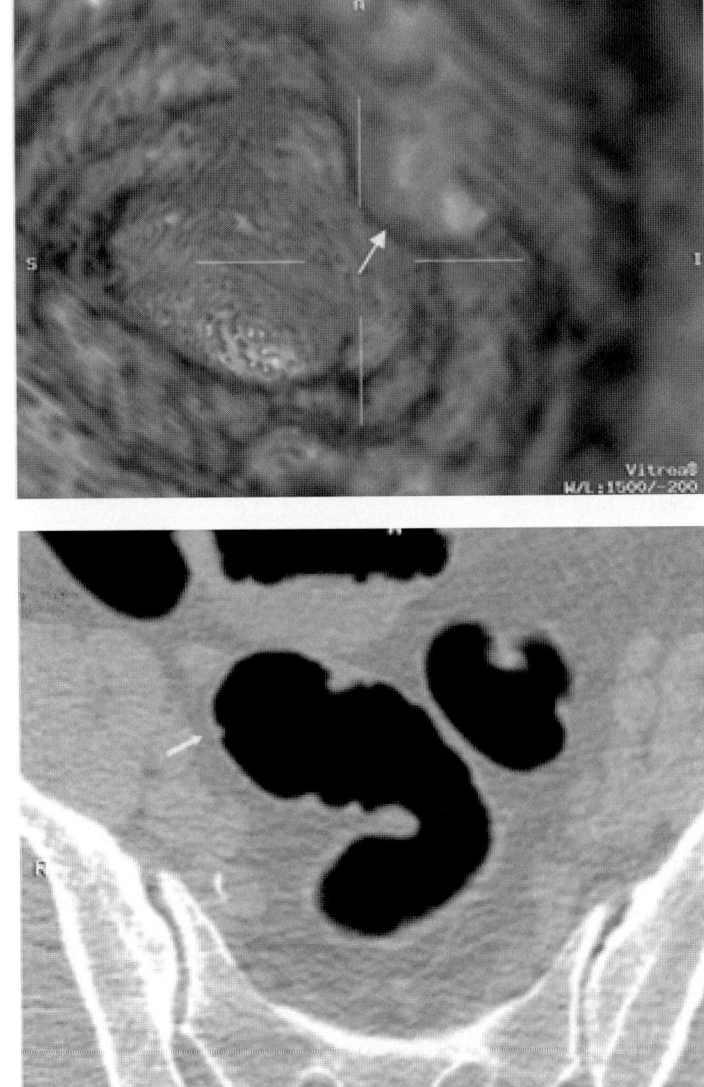

FIGURE 9.1. (*Continued*) (**B**) Corresponding endoluminal view of 9-mm polyp within the sigmoid colon (arrow). (**C**) Transaxial source image.

Continues on next page

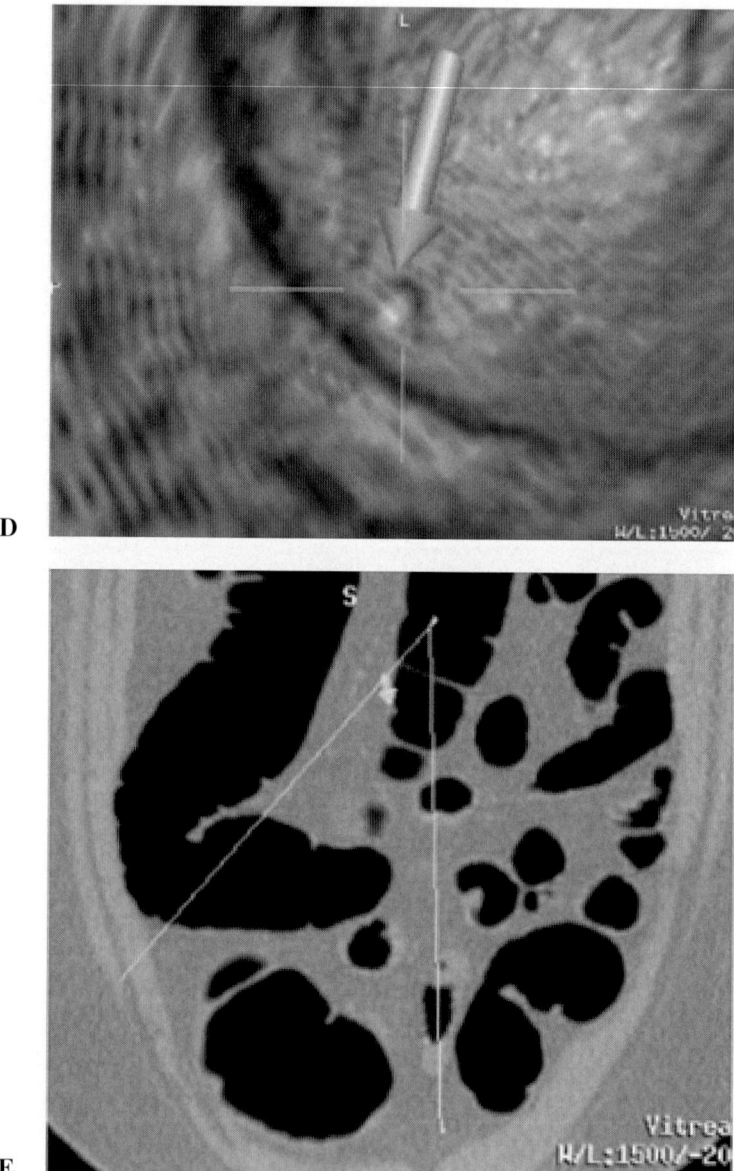

FIGURE 9.1. (*Continued*) (**D**) Corresponding endoluminal view of 3-mm polyp within the sigmoid colon (arrow). (**E**) Coronal reformation.

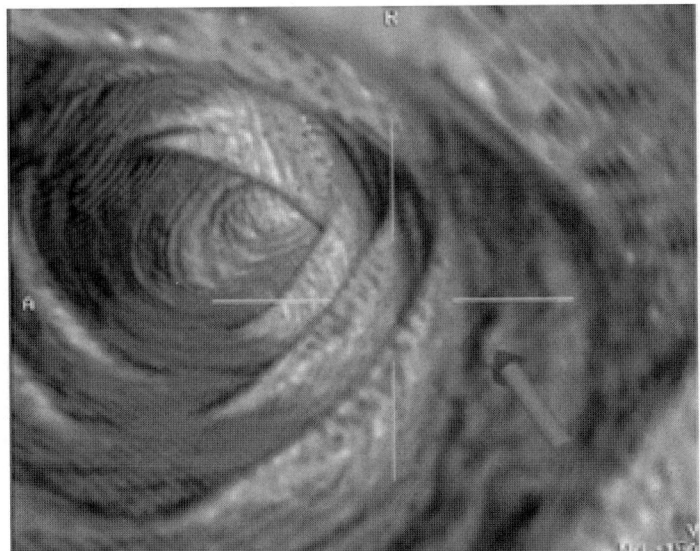

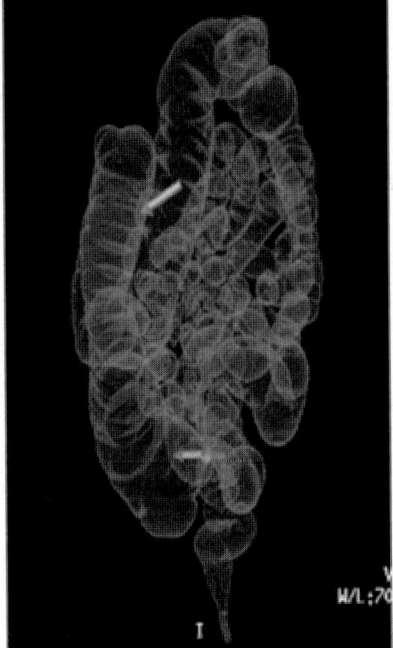

FIGURE 9.1. (*Continued*) (**F**) Corresponding endoluminal view of 3-mm polyp within the transverse colon (arrow). Both 2D MPR and 3D PVR images depict these polyps with great clarity despite increased levels of image noise that result from use of a reduced tube current. (**G**) Edge-enhanced extraluminal volume rendering, with increased transparency, permits visualization of arrows embedded in the 3D volume that indicate the position of these three polyps. Anatomic detail is well preserved despite relatively high levels of image noise.

Conclusion

Although a variety of techniques are available for performing CTC, it is important to ensure that high levels of diagnostic accuracy are achieved without exposing patients to excessive radiation. Thin-section examination with either SDCT or MDCT should be accompanied by a limitation in x-ray tube current to keep radiation dose equivalent to or less than the dose imparted with an air–contrast barium enema. This necessarily requires an increase in image noise, which should be acceptable for detection of colonic polyps in an air-filled lumen. At the same time, such levels of image noise may not be acceptable for detection of incidental or ancillary findings, which rely on low-contrast detectability, such as subtle lesions within the liver. Although increasing pitch will reduce dose with SDCT colonography, the same is not necessarily true for MDCT colonography. Most MDCT manufacturers automatically increase tube current to produce equal noise when pitch is increased (Mahesh et al. 2001). Radiation dose will be lowered only if this feature is manually overridden. As such, low-dose, high-resolution CTC requires diligence and concern on the part of both the technologist and radiologist alike.

References

Ahlquist DA, Wieland HS, Moertel CG, et al. Accuracy of fecal occult blood screening for colorectal neoplasia. A prospective study using Hemoccult and HemoQuant tests. JAMA 1993;269:1262–1267.

Beaulieu CF, Jeffrey RB, Jr, Karadi C, et al. Display modes for CT colonography. Part II. Blinded comparison of axial CT and virtual endoscopic and panoramic endoscopic volume-rendered studies. Radiology 1999;212(1):203–212.

Beaulieu CF, Napel S, Daniel BL, et al. Detection of colonic polyps in a phantom model: Implications for virtual colonoscopy data acquisition. J Comput Assist Tomogr 1998;22:656–663.

Blackstone MO. The colon-endoscopic orientation, technique of examination, and normal appearance. In: Blackstone MO, ed. Endoscopic Interpretation—Normal and Pathologic Appearances of the Gastrointestinal Tract. New York: Raven Press; 1984:401–427.

Brown ML, Thompson GB, Kessler LG. The knowledge and use of screening tests for colorectal and prostate cancer: Data from the 1987 National Health Interview Survey. 1990; Prev Med 19:562–574.

Byers T, Levin B, Rothenberger D, Dodd GD, Smith RA. American Cancer Society guidelines for screening and surveillance for early detection of colorectal polyps and cancer: Update 1997. CA Cancer J Clin 1997;47:154–160.

Callstrom MR, Johnson CD, Fletcher JG, et al. CT colonography without cathartic preparation: Feasibility study. Radiology 2001;219:693–698.

Chan HP, Sahiner B, Helvie MA, et al. Improvement of radiologists' characterization of mammographic masses by using computer-aided diagnosis: An ROC study. Radiology 1999;212:817–827.

Chen D, Liang Z, Wax MR, Li L, Li B, Kaufman AE. A novel approach to extract colon lumen from CT images for virtual colonoscopy. IEEE Trans Med Imag 2000;19:1220–1226.

Chen SC, Lu DSK, Hecht JR, Ladell BM. CT colonography: Value of scanning in both the supine and prone positions. JR 1999;172:595–600.

Cline HE, Dumoulin CL, Hart HR, et al. 3D reconstruction of the brain from magnetic resonance images using a connectivity algorithm. Magnet Reson Imag 1987;5(5):345–352.

Dachman AH, Diagnostic performance of virtual colonoscopy Abdom Imaging 2002;27:260–267.

Dachman AH, Kuniyoshi JK, Boyle CM, et al. CT colonography with three-dimensional problem solving for detection of colonic polyps. AJR 1998;171:989–995.

Dave SB, Wang G, Brown BP, et al. Straightening the colon with curved cross sections: An approach to CT colonography. Acad Radiol 1999;6(7):398–410.

Day DW, Morson BC. The adenoma–carcinoma sequence. In: Morson BC, ed. The Pathogenesis of Colorectal Cancer. Philadelphia: WS Saunders Co; 1978:58–71.

Debatin JF, Lubolt W, Baverfeind P. Virtual colonoscopy in 1999: computed tomography or magnetic resonance imaging? Endoscopy 1999;31:174–179.

Elwood MJ, Ali G, Schlup MT, et al. Flexible sigmoidoscopy or colonoscopy for colorectal screening: A randomized trial of performance and acceptability. Cancer Detect Prevent 1995;19:337–347.

Fenlon HM, Clarke PD, Ferrucci JT. Virtual colonoscopy: Imaging features with colonoscopic correlation. AJR 1998;170:1303–1309.

Fenlon HM, Ferrucci JT. Virtual colonoscopy: What will the issues be? AJR 1997;169: 453–458.

Fenlon HM, Ferrucci JT. First international symposium on virtual colonoscopy. AJR 1999;173:565–569. (a)

Fenlon HM, Nunes DP, Schroy PC, et al. A comparison of virtual and conventional colonoscopy for the detection of colorectal polyps. N Engl J Med 1999;341:1496–1503. (b)

Fletcher JG, Luboldt W. CT colonography and MR colonography: Current status, research directions, and comparison. Eur Radiol 2000;10:786–801.

Fletcher JG, Johnson CD, Welch TJ, MacCarty RL, Ahlquist DA, Reed JE, Harmsen WS, Wilson LA. Optimization of CT colonography technique: Prospective trial in 180 patients. Radiology 2000;216:704–711.

Frommer DJ. What's new in colorectal cancer screening? J Gastroenterol Hepatol 1998;13: 528–533.

Glick S. Double-contrast barium enema for colorectal cancer screening: A review of the issues and a comparison with other screening alternatives. AJR 2000;174:1529–1537.

Glick S, Wagner JL, Johnson CD. Cost-effectiveness of double contrast barium enema in screening for colorectal cancer. AJR 1998;170:629–636.

Gokturk SB, Tomas C, Acar B, et al. A statistical 3-D pattern processing method for computer-aided detection of polyps in CT colonography. IEEE Trans Med Imag 2001; 20:1251–1260.

Griswold MA, Jakob PM, Nittka M, Goldfarb JW, Haase A. Partially parallel imaging with localized sensitivities (PILS). Magn Reson Med 2000;44:602–609.

Hara AK, Johnson CD, Reed JE, Ehman JE, Ilstrup DM. Colorectal polyp detection with CT colonography: Two- versus three-dimensional techniques. Radiology 1996;200:49–54.

Hara AK, Johnson CD, Reed JE, et al. Reducing data size and radiation dose for CT colonography. AJR 1997;168:1181–1184.

Johnson CD, Dachman AH. CT colonography: The next colon screening examination. Radiology 2000;216:331–341.

Johnson PI, Heath HG, Bliss DF, et al. Three-dimensional CT: Real-time interactive volume rendering. Radiology 1996;200:581–583.

Kobayashi T, Xu XW, MacMahon H, Metz CE, Doi K. Effect of a computer-aided diagnosis scheme on radiologists' performance in detection of lung nodules on radiographs. Radiology 1996;199:843–848.

Lauenstein TC, Goehde SC, Ruehm SG, et al. MR colonography with barium-based fecal tagging: Initial clinical experience. Radiology 2002;223:248–254.

Lauenstein TC, Holtmann G, Schoenfelder D, et al. MR colonography without bowel cleansing: A new strategy to improve patient acceptance. AJR 2001;177:823–827.

Lomas DJ, Sood RR, Graves MJ, Miller R, Hall NR, Dixon AK. Colon carcinoma: MR imaging with CO_2 enema. Radiology 2001;219:558–562.

Lorensen WE, Cline HE. Marching cubes: A high-resolution 3D surface reconstruction system. Comput Graph 1987;21:163–169.

Lorensen WE, Jolesz FA, Kikinis R. The exploration of cross-sectional data with a virtual endoscope. In: Interactive Technology and the New Paradigm for Health Care: Medicine Meets Virtual Reality III Proceedings. Amsterdam: IOS Press; 1995.

Luboldt W, Bauerfeind P, Steiner P, et al. Preliminary assessment of three-dimensional magnetic resonance imaging for various colonic disorders. Lancet 1997;349:1288–1291.

Luboldt W, Bauerfeind P, Wildermuth S, et al. Colonic masses: Detection with MR colonography. Radiology 2000;216:383–388.

Luboldt W, Steiner P, Bauerfeind P, Pelkonen P, Debatin JF. Detection of mass lesions with MR colonography. Radiology 1998;207:59–65.

Macari M, Berman P, Dicker M, Milano A, Megibow A. Usefulness of CT colonography in patients with incomplete colonography. AJR 1999;173:561–564.

Macari M, Bini E, Milano A, Katz S, Resnick BS, Megibow AJ. Low-dose CT colonography in colorectal polyp detection. Radiology 2001;221(P):403. (a)

Macari M, Bini EJ, Xue X, Milano A, Katz S, Resnick D, Chandarana H, Klingenbeck K, Krinsky G, Marshall CH, Megibow AJ. Prospective comparison of thin-section low-dose multislice CT colonography to conventional colonoscopy in detecting colorectal polyps and cancers. Radiology 2002;224:383–392.

Macari M, Megibow AJ. Pitfalls using 3D CT colonography with 2D imaging correlation. AJR 2001;176:137–143. (b)

Macari M, Milano A, Lavelle M, Berman P, Megibow AJ. Comparison of time-efficient CT colonography with two- and three-dimensional colonic evaluation for detecting colorectal polyps. AJR 2000;174:1543–1549.

Macari M, Pedrosa I, Lavelle M, Milano A, Dicker M, Megibow AJ, Xue X. Effect of different bowel preparations on residual fluid at CT colonography. Radiology 2001;218: 274–277. (c)

Mahesh M, Scatarige JC, Cooper J, Fishman EK. Dose and pitch relationship for a particular multislice CT scanner. AJR 2001;177:1273–1275.

Mandel JS, Bond JH, Church TR, et al. Reducing mortality from colorectal cancer by screening for fecal occult blood. N Engl J Med 1993;328:1365–1371.

Marcos HB, Semelka RC. Evaluation of Crohn's disease using half-fourier RARE and gadolinium-enhanced SGE sequences: Initial results. Magn Reson Imag 2000;18:263–268.

Masutani Y, Yoshida H, MacEneaney P, Dachman A. Automated segmentation of colonic walls for computerized detection of polyps in CT colonography. J Comput Assist Tomogr 2001;25:629–638.

McCollough CH, Zink FE. Performance evaluation of a multi-slice CT system. Med Phys 1999;26:2223–2230.

McDermott RA, McFarland EG, Brink JA, Ristvedt SL, Menias CO, Littenberg B, et al. Prospective comparison of air and CO2 insufflation techniques at CT colonography: Evaluation of image quality and patient reactions. Radiology 2001;221(P):578.

McFarland EG, Brink JA, Heiken JP, Balfe DM, Hirselj D, Pilgram TK, Weinstock L, Littenberg. Spiral CT colonography: Reader reliability and diagnostic performance with 2D and 3D image displays. Radiology 2000;218:375–383.

McFarland EG, Brink JA, Loh J, Wang G, Argiro V, et al. Visualization of colorectal polyps with spiral CT colonography: Evaluation of processing parameters with perspective volume rendering. Radiology 1997;205:701–707.

McFarland EG, Brink JA, Pilgram TK, et al. Spiral CT colonography: Reader agreement and diagnostic performance with two- and three-dimensional image-display techniques. Radiology 2001;218:375–383.

McFarland E. Reader strategies for CT colonography. Abdom Imaging 2002;27:275–283.

McFarland EG. Pilgram TK, Brink JA, McDermott RA, Santillan CV, Brady PW, et al, Multi-observer diagnostic performance of CT colonography: factors influencing diagnostic-accuracy assessment. Radiology 2002 (in press).

Metz CE. Evaluation of CAD methods. In: Hoffmann KR, ed. Computer-Aided Diagnosis in Medical Imaging. Amsterdam: Elsevier Science; 1999;543–554.

Morrin MM, Kruskal JB, Farrell RJ, Goldberg SN, McGee JB, Raptopoulos V. Endoluminal CT colonography after an incomplete endoscopic colonoscopy. AJR 1999;172: 913–918.

Morrin MM, Farrell RJ, Kruskal JB, Reynolds K, McGee JB, Raptopoulos V. Utility of intravenously administered contrast material at CT colonography. Radiology 2000;217: 765–771.

Morrin MM, Hochman MG, Farrell RJ, Marquesuzaa H, Rosenberg S, Edelman RR. MR colonography using colonic distention with air as the contrast material. AJR 2001;176: 144–146.

Morrin MM, Kruskal JB, Ferrell RJ, Reynolds KF, Raptopoulos VD. Does glucagon improve colonic distention and polyp detection during CT colonography? Radiology 1999;213(Suppl):341. Abstract.

Napel S, Rubin GD, Jeffrey RB. STS-MIP: A new reconstruction technique for CT of the chest. J Comput Assist Tomogr 1993;17:832–838.

Nappi J, Yoshida H. Automated detection of polyps in CT colonography: Evaluation of volumetric features for reduction of false positives. Acad Radiol 2002;22:963–979.

Neuhaus H. Screening for colorectal cancer in Germany: Guidelines and reality. Endoscopy 1999;31:468–470.

O'Brien MJ, Winawer SJ, Zauber AG, Gottlieb LS, Sternberg SS, Diaz B, Dickersin GR, Ewing S, Geller S, Kasimian D. The National Polyp Study. Patient and polyp characteristics associated with high-grade dysplasia in colorectal adenomas. Gastroenterology 1990;98:371–379.

Paik DS, Beaulieu CF, Jeffrey RB, et al. Automated flight path planning for virtual endoscopy. Med Phys 1998;25(5):629–637.

Paik DS, Beaulieu CF, Jeffrey RB Jr, et al. Visualization modes for CT colonography using cylindrical and planar map projections. J Comput Assist Tomogr 2000;24:179–188.

Paik DS, Beaulieu CF, Jeffrey RB, Karadi C, Napel S. Detection of polyps in CT colonography: A comparison of a computer-aided detection algorithm to 3D visualization methods. Radiology 1999;213P:197.

Pappalardo G, Polettini E, Frattaroli FM, et al. Magnetic resonance colonography versus conventional colonoscopy for the detection of colonic endoluminal lesions. Gastroenterology 2000;119:300–304.

Pescatore P, Glucker T, Delarive J, Meuli R, Pantoflickova D, Duvoisin B, Schnyder P, Blum AL, Dorta G. Diagnostic accuracy and interobserver agreement of CT colonography (virtual colono-scopy). Gut 2000;47:126–130.

Read TE, Read JD, Butterly FL. Importance of adenomas 5 mm or less in diameter that are detected by sigmoidoscopy. N Engl J Med 1997;336:8–12.

Reed JE, Johnson CD. Automatic segmentation, tissue characterization, and rapid diagnosis enhancements to the computed tomographic colonography analysis workstation. J Digit Imag 1997;10(3, Suppl 1):70–73.

Reed JE, Johnson CD. Virtual pathology: A new paradigm for interpretation of computed tomographic colonography. In: Kim Y, Mun SK, eds. Medical Imaging 1998: Image Display. vol 3335. Bellingham, Wash: International Society of Optic Engineering, 1998: 439–449.

Rex DK, Cummings OW. The controversy regarding distal hyperplastic polyps. Gastrointest Endo Clin North Am 1993;3:639–649.

Rex DK, Cutler CS, Lemmel GT, et al. Colonoscopic miss rates of adenomas determined by back-to-back colonoscopies. Gastroenterology 1997;112:24–28.

Robinson AH. Elements of Cartography. 6th ed. New York: Wiley; 1995.

Rogalla P, Bender A, Bick U, et al. Tissue transition projection (TTP) of the intestines. Eur Radiol 2000;10:806–810.

Royster AP, Fenlon HM, Clarke PD, et al. CT colonoscopy of colorectal neoplasms: Two dimensional and three dimensional virtual reality techniques with colonoscopic correlation. AJR 1997;169:1237–1242.

Rubin GD, Beaulieu CF, Argiro V, et al. Perspective volume rendering of CT and MR images: Applications for endoscopic imaging. Radiology 1996;199:321–330.

Saar B, Heverhagen JT, Obst T, et al. Magnetic resonance colonography and virtual magnetic resonance colonoscopy with the 1.0-T system: A feasibility study. Invest Radiol 2000;35:521–526.

Samara Y, Fiebich M, Dachman AH, et al. Automated calculation of the centerline of the human colon on CT images. Acad Radiol 1999;6:352–359.

Selby JV, Friedman GD, Quesenberry CP, Weiss NS. A case-control study of screening sigmoidoscopy and mortality from colorectal cancer. N Engl J Med 1992;326:653–657.

Sheikh S, Paik DS, Beaulieu CF, et al. Wide-Angle Virtual Endoscopy with Multiple-View Rendering: The Virtual Cockpit. RSNA-EJ. http://ej.rsna.org/ej2/0085-98.fin/vc/virtual-cockpit.html. 1998.

Snyder JP. Flattening the Earth: Two Thousand Years of Map Projections. Chicago: University of Chicago Press; 1993.

Springer P, Stohr B, Giacomuzzi SM, et al. Virtual computed tomography colonoscopy: Artifacts, image quality, and radiation dose load in a cadaver study. Eur Radiol 2000;10:183–187.

Spinzi G, Belloni G, Martegani A, Sangiovanni A, Del Favero C, Minoli G. Computed tomographic colonography and conventional colonoscopy for colon diseases: A prospective, blinded study. Am J Gastroenterol 2001;96:394–400.

Summers RM. Morphometric methods for virtual endoscopy reconstructions. In: Bankman IN, ed. Handbook of Medical Imaging: Processing and Analysis. San Diego: Academic; 2000;747–755. (a)

Summers RM. Challenges for computer-aided diagnosis for CT colonography. Abdom Radiol 2002;27:268–274.

Summers RM, Beaulieu CF, Pusanik LM, Malley JD, Jeffrey RB, Glazer DI, Napel S. Automated polyp detector for CT colonography: Feasibility study. Radiology 2000;216: 284–290. (b)

Summers RM, Hara AK, Luboldt W, Johnson CD. Computed tomographic and magnetic resonance colonography: Summary of progress from 1995 to 2000. Curr Probl Diagnost Radiol 2001;30:141–168. (a)

Summers RM, Jerebko AK, Franaszek M, Malley JD. An integrated system for computer-aided diagnosis in CT colonography: Work-in-progress. In: Computer Assisted Radiology and Surgery (CARS). Berlin: Elsevier Science; 2001:629–634. (b)

Summers RM, Johnson CD, Pusanik LM, et al. Automated polyp detection at CT colonography: Feasibility assessment in a human population. Radiology 2001;219:51–59. (c)

Summers RM, Pusanik LM, Malley JD. Automatic detection of endobronchial lesions with virtual bronchoscopy: Comparison of two methods. In: Medical Imaging 1998: Image Processing. San Diego: SPIE; 1998(3338):327–335.

Summers RM, Pusanik LM, Malley JD, Reed JE, Johnson CD. Method of labeling colonic polyps at CT colonography using computer-assisted detection. In: Computer Assisted Radiology and Surgery (CARS). San Francisco: Elsevier Science; 2000:785–789. (a)

Summers RM, Selbie WS, Malley JD, et al. Polypoid lesions of airways: Early experience with computer-assisted detection by using virtual bronchoscopy and surface curvature. Radiology 1998;208:331–337. (b)

Svensson MH, Svensson E, Lasson A, Hellstrom M. Patient acceptance of CT colonography and conventional colonoscopy: Prospective comparative study in patients with or suspected of having colorectal disease. Radiology 2002;222:337–345.

Villavicencio RT, Rex DX. Colonic adenomas: Prevalence and incidence rates, growth rates, and miss rates at colonoscopy. Semn Gastrointest Dis 2000;11:185–193.

Vining DJ, Ge Y, Ahn DK, Stelts DR. Virtual colonoscopy with computer-assisted polyp detection. In: Hoffmann KR, ed. Computer-Aided Diagnosis in Medical Imaging: Proceedings of the First International Workshop on Computer-Aided Diagnosis. Amsterdam: Elsevier Science; 1999:445–452.

Vining DJ, Black TG, Han J. Accuracy of virtual colonography using an oral contrast preparation and controlled gas distension. 27th Annual Scientific Program of the RSNA, Chicago Ill. 2001.

Wang G, McFarland EG, Brown BP, et al. GI tract unraveling with curved cross sections. IEEE Trans Med Imag 1998;17:318–322.

Wax MR, Kreer KA, Anderson J. Endoscopic view in virtual colonoscopy: Achieving complete surface visualization. Radiology 2001;221(P):307. (a)

Wax MR, Bitter I, May S, Wade D, Mazzarese CK. Optimizing bowel preparation for virtual colonoscopy electronic cleansing. Radiology 2001;221(P):578. (b)

Weishaupt D, Patak MA, Fröhlich J, Rühm SG, Debatin JF. Faecal tagging to avoid colonic cleaning before MRI colonography. Lancet 1999;354:835–836.

Weitzman: Risk and reluctance: Understanding impediments to colorectal cancer screening. Prev Med 2001;32.

Winawer SJ, Fletcher RH, Miller L, et al. Colorectal cancer screening: Clinical guidelines and rationale. Gastroenterology 1997;112:594–642.

Winawer SJ, Zauber AG, Ho MN, et al. Prevention of colorectal cancer by colonoscopic polypectomy. N Engl J MEd 1993;329:1977–1981.

Yee J, Akerkar GA, Hung RK, Steinauer-Gebauer AM, Wall SD, McQuaid KR. Colorectal neoplasia: Performance characteristics of CT colonography for detection in 300 patients. Radiology 2001;219:685–692.

Yee J, Hung RK, Akekar GA, Wall SD. The usefulness of glucagon hydrochloride for colonic distension. AJR 1999;173:169–172. (a)

Yee J, Hung RK, Steinauer-Gebauer AM, Akerkar GA, Wall SD, McQuaid KM. Colonic distention and prospective evaluation of colorectal polyp detection with and without glucagon during CT colonography. Radiology 1999;213(Suppl):256. Abstract. (b)

Yoshida H, Masutani Y, MacEneaney P, Rubin DT, Dachman AH. Computerized detection of colonic polyps at CT colonography on the basis of volumetric features: Pilot study. Radiology 2002;222:327–336. (a)

Yoshida H, Nappi J. Three-dimensional computer-aided diagnosis scheme for detection of colonic polyps. IEEE Trans Med Imag 2001;20:1261–1274.

Yoshida H, Nappi J, MacEneaney P, Rubin DT, Dachman AH. Computer-aided diagnosis scheme for the detection of polyps at CT colonography. RadioGraphics 2002;22:963–979.

Zalis ME, Del Frate C, Hahn PF. Digital subtraction bowel cleansing in CT colonography: Initial experience. 86th Annual Scientific Paper RSNA, Chicago 2000.

Zalis ME, Hahn PF. Digital subtraction bowel cleansing in CT colonography. AJR 2001;176:646–648.

Index

A

Accuracy, in computed tomography
    colonography
  cecum, hepatic flexure
    data acquisition, 3D endoluminal, 3D
      endoscopic views, 16–17
    readers, 3D endoluminal, 3D
      endoscopic views, 18
  cecum distention, polyp detection, 3D
    endoluminal view, 17
  data acquisition protocol, 3D
    endoscopic view, 15–18
  hepatic flexure mass, 3D endoscopic
    view, 18
  image display, coronal, 3D endoscopic
    views, 16–17
  overview, 14–23
    interobserver agreement, using
      different image display techniques,
      22
    study parameters, 14–18
    three-dimensional interpretation,
      18–21
    two-dimensional interpretation, 18–21
    validation, future areas of, 22–23
  patient selection, 14
  sigmoid polyp, 2D view, 3D view
    compared, 16–17
  sigmoid polyp image display, 16
Adenocarcinoma, partially constricting,
    3D endoluminal, sagittal views, 40
Adenoma, rectal fold, axial CT, 3D
    endoluminal, compared, 40
Adenomatous polyposis
  future developments, 64

Mercator projection virtual endoscopy,
    60
navigation
  centerline path, 55
  perspective rendering, 53–56,
  panoramic viewing, map projections,
    57–58, 57–61
  panoramic virtual endoscopy, 59
  single-camera virtual endoscopy, 56
    limited visibility of, 57
  slab volume rendering, 63
  three-dimensional display methods,
    53–64
  tissue transition projection, 62
  tomographic colon unraveling, 61–62,
  virtual cockpit, 58
  volume-rendering methods, 62–63
Air, residual, three-dimensional data set
    collection, patient position and, 68
American Cancer Society, screening
    guidelines for colorectal cancer, 8
Ascending colon, polyp, 71

B

Barium sulfate-based fecal tagging, 77
Bowel cleansing, 24–25
  computed tomography colonography, 14
Bowel distention, internal anal sphincter, 27
Bowel preparation, 49–52
  effect of, 87
Bowel wall, thickened, descending colon,
    contrast enhancement, 73
Bright-lumen magnetic resonance
    colonography, 65–70
Bulbous folds, 42–44

C

Cancer
colorectal, screening guidelines for, American Cancer Society, 8
computer-assisted diagnosis, 87–89
obstructing, incomplete coloscopy, 11–12

Cescum
distention, polyp, detection, computed tomography colonography, 3D endoluminal view, 17

Centerline path, navigation, advanced three-dimensional display, 55

Changing window-level settings, prone CT image, narrow W/L settings, descending colon, 36

Cleansing bowel, distention, computed tomography colonography, 14–15

Collapsed colon, endoluminal view of, 39

Colon
ascending polyp, 71
screening for. See Screening, colon cancer
collapsed, endoluminal view of, 39
descending
contrast enhancement, thickened bowel wall, 73
normal, 37–39
sigmoid
polyp-stimulating protrusion, 72
transverse
endoluminal view, 38

Colonic filling, non-slice-selec two-dimensional acquisition collection, 67

Colonic lumen, contrast-filled, surrounding structures, high contrast between, 69

Colonic surface
between folds, diagram, 80
shape, diagram of, computer-aided diagnosis, 80

Colonic wall, folds, polyps, volumetric shape index, differentiation, CT, 3D endoscopic views, 86

Colorectal cancer, screening guidelines for, American Cancer Society, 8

Computed tomography colonography, 14–18
accuracy of, 14–23
interobserver agreement, using different image display techniques, 22
study parameters, 14–18. See Study parameters
three-dimensional interpretation, 18–21
two-dimensional interpretation, 18–21
validation, future areas of, 22–23
colon cancer screening, 10–11

Computed tomography data, management, interpretation of, 30

Computer-aided diagnosis
bowel preparation, effect of, 87–88
in clinical setting, 88
colonic surface shape, diagram of, 80
computer-assisted diagnosis, cancer, 87–89
cost of, 89
future directions, 79–89
image database, 89
polyps, 81
processing time, 89
progress to date, 79–87
scanning parameters, computed tomography, effect of, 88
technical improvements, 88
volumetric shape index polyps, folds, colonic wall, differentiation, CT, 3D endoscopic views, 86

Constricting adenocarcinoma, 3D endoluminal, sagittal views, 40

Contrast-filled colonic lumen, surrounding structures, high contrast between, 69

Conventional colonoscopy, magnetic resonance colonography, compared, 74

Cost, computer-assisted diagnosis, 89

Current screening practices, 9–10

D

Dark-lumen magnetic resonance colonography, 70–74

Data acquisition
patient preparation, 24

protocol, 15–17
  3D endoluminal view, 3D
    endoscopic view, 17
Data interpretation, 35–46
  prone CT image, narrow W/L settings,
    descending colon, 36
Database, image, computer-assisted
  diagnosis, 89
Descending colon, contrast enhancement,
  thickened bowel wall, 73
Diagnostic accuracy, magnetic resonance
  colonography, 74–75
Distention
  bowel, computed tomography
    colonography, 14–15
  cecum, polyp detection, computed
    tomography colonography, 3D
    endoluminal view, 17
Diverticulum, 44
  endoluminal view, 44

E
Endoluminal view
  collapsed colon, 39
  diverticulum, 44
  sigmoid/descending colon junction, 37
  transverse colon, 38
Extrinsic defects, 46

F
Fecal material, residual, 39–42
Fecal tagging, 75–78
  barium sulfate-based, 77
  gadolinium-based, 76
Filing defect, with stool, 41
Fold, polyps, colonic wall, volumetric
  shape index, differentiation, CT,
  3D endoscopic views, 86
Future developments
  in computer-aided diagnosis, 79–89
  in virtual colonoscopy, 3

G
Gadolinium-based fecal tagging, 76

H
Hepatic flexure, mass, computed
  tomography colonography, 3D
  endoscopic view, 18

Historical perspective, colon cancer
  screening, 4–9
Hypotonia, 25–26

I
Ileocecal valve, 3D endoluminal, coronal
  CT, 44–45
Incomplete colonoscopy, 11–12
  obstructing cancer, 11–12
Initiation of exam, 25
Insufflation, 26
Interobserver agreement, computed
  tomography colonography, using
  different image display techniques,
  22
Interpretation of VC exam, 24–46
  computed tomography data, 30
  data interpretation, 35–46
    prone, supine, wide W/L setting,
    narrow W/L setting, 35
    prone CT image, narrow W/L
    settings, descending colon, 36
  diverticulum, endoluminal view, 44
  endoluminal view, sigmoid/descending
    colon junction, 37
  fecal material, residual, 39–42
  fluid, positioning, redistribution of,
    prone CT image, narrow W/L
    settings, descending colon, 35
  future developments, 46

M
Magnetic resonance colonography, 65–78
  ascending colon, polyp, 71
  barium sulfate-based fecal tagging, 77
  bright-lumen, 65–70
  colonic filling, two-dimensional
    acquisition collection, 67
  colonic lumen, contrast-filled,
    surrounding structures, high
    contrast between, 69
  conventional colonoscopy, compared
    to, 74
  dark-lumen, 70–74
  descending colon, contrast
    enhancement, thickened bowel
    wall, 73
  diagnostic accuracy, 74–75
  fecal tagging, 75–78

Magnetic resonance colonography
    (*continued*)
    gadolinium-based fecal tagging, 76
    polyp-stimulating protrusion, sigmoid
        colon, 72
    residual air, three-dimensional dataset
        collection, patient position and, 68
    technique, 65–74
    three-dimensional GRE data set,
        maximum intensity projection, 68
    without fecal tagging, without prior
        bowel cleansing, 77
Map projections, panoramic viewing,
        advanced three-dimensional
        display, 57–61
Mercator projection virtual endoscopy, 41
Mobile filing defect, with stool, 41
Multiplanar reconstructions, value of,
        rectum, axial CT, # 3D
        endoluminal, compared, axial CT,
        coronal image, compared, 33

N
Navigation
    centerline path, advanced three-
        dimensional display, 55
    perspective rendering, advanced three-
        dimensional display, 53–56

O
Obstructing cancer, incomplete
        colonoscopy, 11–12

P
Panoramic viewing, map projections,
        advanced three-dimensional
        display, 57–61
Panoramic virtual endoscopy, 59
Patient education, 47–49
Patient position, residual air, three-
        dimensional dataset collection, 68
Patient preparation, 47–52
    bowel preparation, 49–52
    data acquisition, 24
    patient education, 47–49
Patient selection, computed tomography
        colonography, 14
Performance, interpretation of VC exam,
        24–46
    adenocarcinoma, partially constricting,
        3D endoluminal, sagittal views, 40

bowel cleansing, 24–25
bowel distention, internal anal
        sphincter, 27
bulbous folds, 42–44
colon
    collapsed, endoluminal view of, 39
    normal, 37–39
    transverse, endoluminal view, 38
computed tomography data,
        management, interpretation of,
        30
data interpretation, 35–46
    prone CT image, narrow W/L
        settings, descending colon, 36
diverticulum, 44
    endoluminal view, 44–45
endoluminal view, sigmoid/descending
        colon junction, 37
extrinsic defects, 46
fecal material, residual, 39–42
fluid, positioning, redistribution of,
        prone CT image, narrow W/L
        settings, descending colon, 36
future developments, 46
hypotonia, 25–26
ileocecal valve, 3D endoluminal,
        coronal CT, 44–45
initiation of exam, 25
insufflation, 26–27
mobile filing defect, with stool, 41
multiplanar reconstructions, value of,
        rectum, axial CT, 3D endoluminal,
        compared, axial CT, coronal
        image, compared, 33
patient preparation, data acquisition,
        24
preliminary three-dimensional read,
        two-dimensional problem solving
        and, endoluminal view, axial CT
        image, 43
rectum
    fold, with adenoma, axial CT, 3D
        endoluminal, compared, 32
    three-dimensional interpretation,
        axial CT, 3D endoluminal,
        compared, axial CT, coronal
        image, compared, 32–33
    tube, 26
scan performance, 27–28
    internal anal sphincter, 27

slice thickness, effect on image quality,
descending colon, axial CT, 3D
endoluminal, compared, 29
technical scan parameters, 28–29
descending colon, axial CT, 3D
endoluminal, compared, 29
three-dimensional interpretation, 32–35
two-dimensional interpretation, 30–32
window-level settings, changing, prone
CT image, narrow W/L settings,
descending colon, 36
Perspective rendering, navigation,
advanced three-dimensional
display, 53–57
Polyp
ascending colon, 71
computer-aided diagnosis, 81
detection of, cecum distention,
computed tomography
colonography, 3D endoluminal
view, 17
diagram, 80
flat, folds, colonic wall, volumetric
shape index, differentiation, CT,
3D endoscopic views, 86
sigmoid, computed tomography
colonography, study parameters,
2D view, 3D view compared,
16–17
Polyp-stimulating protrusion, sigmoid
colon, 72
Positioning fluid, window-level settings,
changing, prone CT image, narrow
W/L settings, descending colon, 36
Preparation of bowel, 49–52
Processing time, computer-assisted
diagnosis, 89

R
Radiation dose, 90–98
Readers, computed tomography
colonography, 18
cecum, hepatic flexure, 3D endoluminal
view, 3D endoscopic view, 18
Rectum
fold, with adenoma, axial CT, 3D
endoluminal, compared, 32
tube, 26
Residual air, three-dimensional dataset
collection, patient position and, 68

S
Scan performance, 27–28
internal anal sphincter, 27
Scanning parameters, computed
tomography, effect of, 88
Screening
colon cancer
computed tomography colonography,
10–11
historical perspective, 4–9
current practices, 9–10
guidelines for colorectal cancer,
American Cancer Society, 8
Sigmoid colon
polyp, computed tomography
colonography, 2D view, 3D view,
compared, 16–17
polyp-stimulating protrusion, 72
Sigmoid/descending colon junction,
endoluminal view, 37
Single-camera virtual endoscopy
advanced three-dimensional display,
56
limited visibility of, advanced three-
dimensional display, 57
Slab volume rendering, 63
Slice thickness
effect on image quality, descending
colon, axial CT, 3D endoluminal,
compared, 29
Stool, filing defect with, 41
Study parameters, accuracy of computed
tomography colonography, 15–16
bowel cleansing, distention, 14–15
cecum distention, polyp detection, 3D
endoluminal view, 17
data acquisition protocol, 15
cecum, hepatic flexure, 3D
endoluminal view, 3D endoscopic
view, 17–18
hepatic flexure mass, 3D endoscopic
view, 18
image display, sigmoid polyp, 2D view,
3D view, compared, 16
patient selection, 14
readers, cecum, hepatic flexure, 3D
endoluminal view, 3D endoscopic
view, 18
sigmoid polyp, # 2D view, 3D view,
compared, 16–17

T
Tagging, fecal, 75–78
  barium sulfate-based, 77
  gadolinium-based, 76
Technical improvements, computer-aided
    diagnosis, 87–89
Technical scan parameters
  descending colon, axial CT, 3D
      endoluminal, compared, 29
Thickness, slice, effect on image quality,
    descending colon, axial CT, 3D
    endoluminal, compared, 29
Three-dimensional data set collection,
    residual air, patient position and,
    68
Three-dimensional display methods,
    advanced, 53–64
  future developments, 64
  Mercator projection virtual endoscopy,
    60
  navigation
    centerline path, 55
    perspective rendering, 53–56
  panoramic viewing, map projections,
    57–61
  panoramic virtual endoscopy, 59
  single-camera virtual endoscopy, 56
    limited visibility of, 57
  slab volume rendering, 63
  tissue transition projection, 62
  tomographic colon unraveling, 61–62
  virtual cockpit, 58
  volume-rendering methods, 62–63
Three-dimensional GRE data set,
    maximum intensity projection, 68
Three-dimensional interpretation, 34–35
  computed tomography colonography,
    18–21

  preliminary, two-dimensional problem
      solving and, endoluminal view,
      axial CT image, 43
  rectum, axial CT, 3D endoluminal,
      compared, axial CT, coronal
      image, compared, 32–33
Tissue transition projection, 62
Tomographic colon unraveling, 61–62
Two-dimensional interpretation, 30–32
  computed tomography colonography,
    18–21

V
Virtual cockpit, advanced three-
    dimensional display, 58
Virtual colonoscopy, future developments
    in, 3
Visibility, limited, single-camera virtual
    endoscopy, advanced three-
    dimensional display, 57
Volume-rendering methods, advanced
    three-dimensional display, 62–63
Volumetric shape index
  polyps, folds, colonic wall,
      differentiation, CT, 3D endoscopic
      views, 86
  shape classes, relationship between,
      CT, 3D endoscopic views, 85

W
Wide-angle view, three-dimensional
    display methods, virtual cockpit,
    58
Window-level settings, changing, wide
    W/L setting, narrow W/L setting,
    36